OUR CHOICES MATTER

OUR CHOICES MATTER

A Simple Guide to Optimize Health

S. T. GARDNER

OUR CHOICES MATTER
A Simple Guide to Optimize Health

Cover design by Elizabeth T. Gardner.

This book is dedicated to Steve, Elizabeth, and Emily.

ISBN: 979 8 36397 138 9 (paperback)
ISBN: 979 8 37843 884 6 (hardcover)
Imprint: Independently Published

CONTENTS

Preface

I did not research health and nutrition for the purpose of writing a book. I wanted to learn more about the conflicting advice that currently exists in this field. In my attempt to improve my health and the health of my family, I discovered important information that needed to be to be shared. I learned that we have the ability to stay healthy and reduce our chances of getting chronic diseases. We need to be aware of how our current food environment and the lack of crucial information are negatively affecting us. With this understanding we can make better choices to maintain or improve our health.

Our current healthcare system and pharmaceutical industry are not serving us as they should. Because of the way the system is set up, managed, and regulated, they are not equipped with tools or incentives to help keep people healthy but instead can only concentrate on treating symptoms and illnesses.

It has been believed for too long that medical and pharmaceutical science is the answer to human health. It is not. We have neglected to focus on the most powerful tool we have to heal. It is our own amazing bodies. By working with what our bodies need, like proper food and lifestyle, we can heal and thrive. It is empowering to know that we can save ourselves from unintentional self-inflicted harm and stay out of the medication based health system that may make it harder for us to heal. I hope that I can make a difference and encourage people to look at health differently, see the big picture, and understand how our environment has been and is still affecting us. Optimal health is possible, but we have to see beyond the misinformation and make some changes to our food choices and lifestyle.

Human health and nutrition science continually evolves. Our current understanding based on previous research or current science should never be assumed to be infallible. That is how science progresses in any field. New credible data can provide us with more questions and debate for better understanding. The influence of preconceived ideas, biases, and the food and pharmaceutical industries' agenda may have contributed to slower progress in this field.

Currently, health advice is full of conflicting facts. For example; fat and cholesterol are bad, fat and cholesterol are good, sugar is bad, sugar is good in moderate amount, all wheat is bad, whole wheat is good, saturated fats are bad, and vegetable oil is heart healthy. I hope to increase your understanding of these conflicted ideas and shed some light on the concept of "calories" as it is used frequently in human health and nutrition.

Nutritional studies on humans can be difficult to conduct and interpret for many reasons. The human body is far more complex than we think it to be. The body includes mechanical, electrical, chemical, and even emotional and spiritual aspects that are yet to be quantified or understood. Ethics, logistics, cost, and time frames involved are valid concerns. Many historical nutritional research or studies were conducted by interviews of specific populations. This observational study method, typically used in epidemiology, can be used to establish some connection between health problems or diseases and possible causes. In cases of food contamination or disease outbreak, this process can be effective but when trying to establish a connection between a certain component of food and health outcome, this method is less effective. Relying on the memory recall of individuals for data, like what the subjects ate for days or months, is not ideal. Even if the recalls were perfect, the results do not prove cause and effect; they provide only correlation. Information inferred from correlation data shouldn't be used to make dietary recommendations to populations because they are not facts but unproven theories. Taking advice from unsubstantiated correlations can have negative unintended consequences.

These observational conclusions have often been misconstrued as facts. For example, the "fact" that dietary cholesterol and saturated fat cause heart disease. This was eventually adopted into government guidelines, which was accepted and propagated by many health agencies. Once this happened, it becomes hard to disagree with or even to question the theory due to the strong biases and political nature of nutrition science. Currently, there is still no hard evidence to confirm that natural dietary fat and cholesterol cause heart disease. In fact, it is the opposite. These are vital substances for healthy heart and brain.

There are conflicts of interest in the field of human nutrition, and pharmaceutical studies. Drawing conclusions from scientific research can be biased based on the design of the study, who is interpreting and who is funding the research. Data manipulation is common. Many credible research results have been unpublished or ignored due to unwanted or unexpected data. This type of research by food manufacturers, the sugar industry, and the pharmaceutical industry has flooded the nutrition and pharmaceutical fields diluting and distracting from actual hard evidence about the harmful effects of sugar, refined grains, and pharmaceuticals.

There is an epidemic of metabolic disorders resulting in high and increasing number of people being diagnosed with insulin resistance, type 2 diabetes, hypertension, fatty liver, obesity, heart disease, and many related illnesses, in developed nations. What was a rare condition fifty years ago is now a worldwide commonality affecting younger populations. Having a chronic metabolic disorder is a major obstacle to having a healthy life or optimal quality of life.

With our recent exposure to COVID-19, it has become more obvious that it is important to maintain our health so that we can overcome the effects of harmful invaders, in this case, a virus. When our metabolic health is impaired, our immune system is also impaired. Looking for vaccines to save us is an option, but we can also work to strengthen our immune system and our total health collectively by keeping a conscious tab of our food choices and lifestyle. This message has not been seriously promoted to us but should be. It is no longer a game of chance when we can stack the odds in our favor.

The book *The Complete Guide to Fasting* by Jason Fung, MD, was an eye opener for me. Dr. Fung is a nephrologist who treated numerous diabetic patients with failing kidneys and questioned his ineffective methods, sanctioned by what was then the current treatment protocol. He thought outside the box and found a new way to treat his patients by looking at the root cause, not treating the end results. With historical context and information about human biology and survival mechanisms, he observed what was missing in the modern human lifestyle: balance in our time of eating and fasting. The benefits of both are essential for good health.

In *Wheat Belly* by Dr. William Davis, a cardiologist questioned his struggle with weight issues and poor health when he thought he was doing everything right. What he discovered and shared about modern day wheat is mind-boggling. Wheat, including whole grain wheat, and refined flour in large amounts, is generally not good for us. It lacks fiber and nutrients. It is addictive, an appetite stimulant, and can induce mild to severe reaction in those sensitive to certain proteins from the wheat.

In *The Case Against Sugar*, Gary Taubes, an award-winning health and science journalist, presented the compelling cause of chronic diseases to be both sugar (sucrose) and high-fructose corn syrup (HFCS). Just because sugar has been with us for hundreds of years, does not make it harmless or healthy. It is a long-term addictive toxin. Like tobacco or smoking, sugar in the diet may take ten to twenty years for adverse health conditions to develop. It is the amount, speed, and frequency consumed which has dramatically increased with the availability of soft drinks and processed foods. He is convinced that long-term excess sugar consumption is causing metabolic disorders, which include type 2 diabetes, obesity, and heart disease.

Robert Lustig, MD, the author of *Metabolical,* points to processed foods as the culprit to our current health crisis. Processed foods, including sugar, flour, unhealthy trans fats or industrial oils, are harmful in large amounts. Food is healthy if it protects your liver or feeds your gut with fiber and nutrients. Sugar and most processed foods fail this test and should be avoided. It is "what has been done to food" that makes it unhealthy. Whole foods should be consumed as is, or minimally processed. Food can heal or hurt us directly by affecting our complex cellular metabolic processes.

The common wisdom of eating low fat, lean protein, whole grains, and low-calorie diets for better health has been around for decades. The advice is simple enough, so why do more people all over the world have chronic diseases? "Diet and exercise" have been recommended, but many still struggle. Maybe, the advice given is not being followed because it is not convincing enough or maybe few believe it will work. Maybe, the advice is too vague, hard to follow, or not entirely correct.

Many have tried to lose weight based on reducing calorie consumption and exercising more. This method is destined to fail if the calories are not good calories. Limiting calories is not sustainable in the long term and not all calories are equal. The public was already convinced by the "law of thermodynamics" used by the food industry to sell products and unfortunately too, by some healthcare professionals. General wisdom still recommends taking in fewer calories and expending more energy will result in weight loss. This may be true in some cases, but not when the calories consumed are from sugar and refined grains. Our bodies respond to food not calories. Due to the complexity of the body, especially how it senses nutrients, releases certain hormones, and adjusts metabolism to regulate weight and fat accumulation; just controlling calorie input or output is not the way to optimize health or to change your weight.

Type 2 diabetes is generally considered to be a progressive disease, not curable, and can be treated by controlling blood glucose level with medication or insulin. This chronic disease can be progressive and debilitating. Blindness, organ failures, or limb amputation may result before death as a result of poor blood sugar control. It is also true that many have reversed and cured themselves of this condition with food and lifestyle changes. This information should make us think about our current treatment protocol. Many times, when patients are diagnosed with type 2 diabetes, they are often advised to manage their condition with drugs or insulin. Assumption is made by many who are being diagnosed each day and sadly too by many healthcare professionals that this disease is incurable. The current treatment with the advice, eat healthier, exercise, and take your medication may work for a few, but is not a cure for most people. For many, more medication and lower quality of life is in their future.

"Insanity is doing the same thing over and over and expecting different results" quoted by Albert Einstein, applies to our current health recommendation and treatment of chronic metabolic diseases. If our current treatment is not working, as shown by more diagnoses and poor treatment outcomes, we should question the treatment and look for better solutions. If we can find the cause, we should be able to find the cure and prevention. We need to look beyond historical practice, marketing rhetoric, and stubborn common wisdom that are preventing us from seeing how our food environment is affecting us.

Let's not wait until we are already ill to start thinking about our health. Screening for diseases is often part of healthcare. Screening may be good, but a better option is prevention. We have the power to positively influence our health and quality of life. If we know we can make a difference, we will act differently. We should have the facts and the choices.

Introduction

We are not perfect, but our bodies are miracles. Given the right raw materials and conditions, we will heal, adapt, and thrive. Our survival mechanism will prioritize important life-threatening functions over routine functions. Although the human biology is highly complex, our interactions with our bodies are simple.

Modern science has saved and extended lives by helping us heal with medicine, surgery techniques, reduction of deadly infectious diseases, and improving birth mortality. They help with mechanical or chemical interventions, but in the end, our bodies do the healing. Regeneration and repair are inherent to us all, on the surface and at the cellular level.

To most of us, our health span or quality of life matters. Living longer is not the goal, but living with health is. Identifying things that heal and things that harm is the first step in improving or maintaining our quality of life. Many times, it is hard to determine what is which.

Our current food environment and health conditions are intricately linked. It is hard to see the changes in our eating and drinking habits when it happens gradually. Food and nutrition have been taken for granted and assumed to be less important in our daily living. It is usually not included as part of medical care. More focus is placed on the weight of the individual by the amount of calories and fat in the diet. Requiring food producers to provide nutrition label and having fast-food restaurants disclose calorie content in meals may be an attempt to help, but the real problem is still not being recognized because "calorie" is not the problem.

With better information, we can take control of our health. No healthcare professional will care more about you than yourself. Even if they want to help, some may be undereducated about the role of nutrition in health. There is a lifestyle and food choice solution. Because the cure is free, it is not being advertised to us. This solution is simple, but hard to follow in our current environment and "common wisdom" way of thinking.

We are a product of what we eat. Our cells die and regenerate continuously as needed based on where it is located. To have healthy cells, the building blocks of organs and vital systems, we need to have adequate nutrients from food. As part of this regeneration process, there is a cleaning cycle that eliminates dead or impaired cells. We need to let our bodies "clean up" and expel waste materials efficiently. Our metabolic health depends on how our cells use energy and nutrients. Lifestyle and food choices affect these processes.

We share our lives with microorganisms that we are unaware of. They include bacteria, viruses, fungi, and parasites. This collection called microbiome, resides on our skin, in our mouths, and mostly in our intestines. There are more of them than the number of cells in our own bodies, meaning that there is ten times more of their DNA in our bodies than our own. It is within our power to maintain a healthy collection of microbes for our benefit. We need them as much as they need us to survive. By eating well and avoiding toxins, we can cultivate a diverse community of different strains that keep each other in check. It is not "we" against "them," but our mutual survival. The days of fearing germs are gone now that science is learning more about our bodies. There are far more beneficial microbes than harmful ones. The harmful ones have been identified and mitigated by the discovery of antibiotics. These harmful "germs" have given us the fear of all microbes. Eradicating all of them will never happen and should not be our goal. We need to feed our symbiotic "friends" also known as probiotics, with naturally recognizable foods because their survival affects our quality of life.

Manmade sugars (sucrose and high fructose corn syrup (HFCS)) and flour are detrimental to our long-term health.

They are everywhere and are finding more ways to get into our food. Yes, sugar is long-term toxin and flour, a refined grain, is not good for you. We have had sugar and flour in our food supply for hundreds of years. It has been since the past fifty years that the consumption has grown to staggering levels along with the metabolic disorders that follow. It is the amount and frequency. Before the '80s, most people ate three meals a day. Currently, thanks to clever advertisers, most people eat three meals and snacks between all meals, not to mention sugary drinks like sodas, teas, coffees, juices, or sports drinks with each meal or all day long.

Knowing what is good for our bodies is not enough. No amounts of nutritious foods, antioxidants, vitamins, or minerals, will make us healthy if we do not reduce the major source of toxins. Health advice of eating low saturated fats, low calories, and more whole grains has not helped. We need to know what is hurting us. For many people, I believe it is the high frequency and overconsumption of sugar and refined grains (flour).

What is wrong with sugar or flour? And which one of them is less harmful for us? The answers depend on a few factors like lifestyle and genetics, but mostly quantity and frequency of consumption. "The dose makes the poison" quoted by Paracelsus (1493-1541), a Swiss alchemist, known as the father of toxicology, is still true today. Too much of anything, even required substances, can be bad. It is especially true of harmful substances. In general, sugar is more harmful than flour, due to its effect on the liver and production of uric acid. Sugar and flour are often found together in processed foods, cakes, cookies, donuts, cereal, and pastries. These foods, which are associated with celebration and happiness, were historically eaten occasionally, but are now an everyday food. The dose has dramatically increased for the human body, and we have not evolved to process that much in a few generations. Our bodies need food from the earth, and less sugar, flour, and processed foods.

Many blame the obesity epidemic for the cause of increase in numbers of metabolic disorders and type 2 diabetes. It is generally believed that eating too much and not exercising enough will result in obesity. Although this is not entirely correct, it puts the blame on the population and absolves the food and healthcare industries of the burden. It may be true that more overweight people suffer from more chronic metabolic diseases and cancer, but there are overweight individuals who are metabolically healthy and there are thin people with metabolic disorders. Obesity is not the cause but can be one of the many results of metabolic disorders. The metabolic disorder occurs first, which may lead to type 2 diabetes, obesity, chronic inflammation, or other related conditions. Telling the population to lose weight to maintain health is trying to fix a symptom of the problem, not the problem itself. The advice to lose weight is not realistic if the cause of weight gain has not been properly identified. Eating fewer calories may work in the short term for weight reduction, but it is not sustainable, because our bodies need nutrients and energy.

Where our food comes from and how it is grown or processed affects the earth and our health. The commercial agriculture industries have done more harm to our topsoil than we could have imagined. The chemicals in fertilizers, herbicides, and pesticides destroy living organisms in the soil. Without these organisms, soil is just dirt, not able to sustain plant life. A shift to regenerative, sustainable farming is crucial for the survival of future generations. Being aware of the problem is a good first step to finding solutions. The book *Food Fix* by Mark Hyman, MD, provides an insight into problems in our food system and some of the solutions currently being implemented for example composting of food waste and neighborhood gardens.

Fat is necessary for survival. Many functions of fat include, insulation, raw material for cell membranes, processing of fat-soluble vitamins, hormone production, and energy storage. Fat production is automatically regulated to aid survival based on our genetics, diet, and body's needs. Fat is a major energy reserve for possible future famine. It is also how our bodies deal with excess glucose in the blood. Our bodies will take out excess glucose and store them as triglycerides (fat). The easiest way to gain body fat is to eat excess sugar or refined carbohydrates. While fat on the body may be unwanted, fat in our organs like the liver, kidneys, or pancreas, is more dangerous to our health. Many thin people suffer metabolic chronic diseases if their organs have excess fat. It is not always how much fat we are carrying around, but how much and where that fat is located that affects our overall health.

The concept of balancing calorie input and output to adjust weight makes sense until we look at the science. Weight and body composition are not based on calories. Hormones, physical activities, genetics, and the health of our intestines all play a role in determining what our body does with food. Our bodies do not have calorie sensors and do not understand this man-made concept. Some nutritionists and health advisors do not understand this complex process and propagate the "eat less and exercise more" mantra that does not usually help most people loose weight. Balancing energy or calories may be applicable in physics; it does not apply in the same way to biochemistry of the human body. People equate lower calorie intake with health. Food is more than calories; it is nutrients, minerals, and fiber, which are lacking in both sugar and flour. Health is many things including the quality of our mind, blood, organs, and our guts, which are affected by everything we eat. Natural fats, having higher amounts of calories per gram, have been demonized, but in fact, are needed for the brain and heart to function properly. All calories are not equal, so counting them is useless.

It is easier to maintain good health than to have to come back from poor health. Giving up or reducing sugar and refined carbohydrates does not mean giving up the joy of eating delicious foods. With understanding of why we are making these changes, we can enjoy food that is good for us.

Focusing on the healing process by using nutrition and lifestyle to maintain health and heal is part of the emerging preventative and functional medicine, which is needed in healthcare now more than ever. This is not a "diet". It is acknowledging that the body is powerful with healing capabilities and thrives when given the needed resources and environment. Our bodies are resilient and can overcome environmental, physical, and mental trauma, if we find a way to heal by working with, not against it.

We may know people who can eat lots of food, including sugar and flour and are in good health. Very few can get away with it, based on our current worldwide health epidemic. Most people have a tipping point, that when crossed will show symptoms. Some symptoms are physical like metabolic, skin, or digestive conditions. They can also be mental conditions like depression or anxiety. Like lung cancer, metabolic diseases can take up to ten to twenty years to develop. The good news is that lungs will start to heal when smoking is stopped and metabolic diseases can be reversed by better food and lifestyle choices. The bad news is that nicotine addiction is hard to overcome and so is addiction to sugar and flour. What makes it harder is that we know nicotine is not good for us, while very few are acknowledging how harmful and addictive sugar and flour can be.

It is no surprise that food manufacturers are making huge profits and spending millions to keep it that way through marketing, and political influence. They produce foods and drinks that have a long shelf life, so there is less spoilage. They use cheaper ingredients such as, sugar, high fructose corn syrup, refined grains (wheat, corn, soy), and industrial oil, which are all subsidized by our tax dollars (so we pay for it twice when we buy at stores), They hire the best scientists or "cooks" to make their product tasty, addictive, and attractive. They control most of the shelf space available in supermarkets. The best marketing strategies are used to add appeal and create need. Foods are marketed with labels to satisfy our need to be healthy. Food labels are often marked with low fat, low carb, heart healthy, low cholesterol, natural, or high fiber. All this can be meaningless. Look for harmful chemicals, trans fats, and how much sugar was added to assess if it is food or processed chemicals. The goal of the food industry is to sell more products, not to make you healthy.

To be fair, there are a few food companies that are aware of harmful ingredients and are making better products. We need to be more critical of what we buy and eat. Junk food and sodas can be fun once in a while, just not every day. The lines are blurred when trying to decide what food is real or junk. Many ingredients like vitamins, electrolytes, or fiber are added to cereals, breakfast bars, candies, juices, or drinks to entice us further. We need to identify and limit consumption of processed foods. Finding an alternative when convenience is needed due to lack of time, like cereal for breakfast when there is no time for eggs, is logical with the awareness that cereal is a highly processed food and can be full of sugar.

General guidelines for optimizing health:

- Sugar is not essential to the body. There is no essential carbohydrate.
- Whole foods (plant or animal based) including natural fats and cholesterol are essential. We need fatty acids, proteins (amino acids), vitamin, minerals, and fiber. (Trans fats and industrial oils are harmful.)
- Fasting between meals is recommended to maintain sensitivity of the hormone insulin. This hormone is vital for life, but frequent over secretion will have adverse effects on the body.
- Physical movement is vital for your brain and body to function optimally.
- Sleep is vital and should be prioritized.
- Eat sweets and processed foods less often.

- Eating organic, whole food is better for your body and the earth.
- Pain relievers, antibiotics, and medication can be harmful when overused.

People are fed by the food industry, which pays no attention to health, and are healed by the health industry, which pays no attention to food.

- Wendell Berry

1. Food, Nutrition, and Environment

Nature has provided us with many sources of nutrition. Historically, our diets were relatively based on what was available where we lived or settled. Some populations may only have eaten predominantly animal and fish, while other populations may have eaten mostly vegetables, nuts, and roots. Today in the US, we have many available choices. The food industry has provided us with access to countless foods and food products all year long. We rarely think about where our food originated, how it was processed, and how it became available on our store shelves. We marvel at the multitude of products in grocery stores and are unaware of who may have been exploited in this process and what we actually pay for this convenience. The book, *Stuffed and Starved* by Raj Patel is recommended reading for understanding the complex global food system, where small farmers seldom profit compared to large corporations.

We need food to provide us with energy and nutrients. When possible, we should eat real, whole food that is minimally processed and organic. There is no need to count calories. Our ancestors did not count calories or figure out how much carbohydrate, protein, fiber, or fat they were eating. They hunted and gathered to survive. Feast and famine were not unusual. They may have died from infections or many other causes, but not from chronic metabolic diseases. They did not have processed foods or infinite amounts of sugar to consume.

Whole foods contain many varied combinations of macronutrients, known as carbohydrate, protein, fat, and fiber. Also included are micronutrients, such as vitamins, minerals, and phytonutrients. In nature, they are bound together for our benefit and our survival.

Factory processed foods are made by extracting some components of whole foods and refining it so that it has long shelf life for storage and transport. For example, table sugar is the extraction and refining of sugar from sugar canes or sugar beets. Flour is the extraction and refining of wheat, corn, soybeans, or some other plant. It is the refining process that eliminates fiber and nutrients. What is left is powdered carbohydrates. Without nutrients and fibers, they do not spoil. No microorganisms can "eat" it. These ingredients are made in large quantities and are transported to local stores and food factories for further processing.

Crackers, bagels, breads, cookies, muffins, biscuits, chips, cakes, pop tarts, and cereals are examples of foods that can be consistently produced and sold all over the world. These products have long shelf life. They may look and taste good, but are not ideal for frequent consumption. While whole foods provide us with needed energy and nutrients, they have short shelf life and need to be consumed quickly. Processed foods provide mostly energy and very little nutrient. It is the processing that can add preservatives, harmful chemicals, trans fats or industrial oils. Having a diet with mostly processed foods will give you energy, but in excess and long term will impact the function of your liver, pancreas, and may eventually affect your blood glucose control, which leads to many other related chronic diseases.

It is hard to imagine, but it is possible to be overfed and malnourished. This topic is covered in the book *Why We Get Fat* by Gary Taubes. He provided historical data from various regions around the world on the physical effects of poverty on many populations. Obesity and diabetes rates are higher in very poor communities. Diets with mostly flour and sugar, lack of proper nutrition and can result in metabolic dysfunction. Food energy and nutrition are not the same. The human body needs fat, protein, vitamins, minerals, and fiber to function optimally. In these cases, the body may have excess energy (glucose from sugar and flour) the body is starving for nutrients. Native Americans, like the Pima and Sioux, were self-sufficient and healthy until they were relocated to reservations. Their diets transitioned from hunter and gatherer to consuming a modern diet including packaged foods, sodas, and rations of flour and sugar. Within one generation, metabolic diseases became prevalent, where previously were nonexistent. This is true of many indigenous populations that transitioned from their traditional diets to the western modern diet.

When we eat whole foods, either plant or animal based, we don't have to worry about how much fat or cholesterol we are consuming. Fat is satiating and will naturally make us stop eating when we have had enough. Organic meat, whole eggs, seafood, and dairy are nutritious options. They provide protein, essential fatty acids, vitamins, and minerals. Other nutrient dense foods include nuts, seeds, vegetables, fruits, and legumes. When possible, choose vegetables and fruits that are grown organically to reduce exposure to herbicides and pesticides. Locally grown produce supports local farmers and reduce the environmental impact of transportation. Whole plants also provide healthy complex carbohydrates with soluble and insoluble fiber, which are needed to maintain gut health.

Industrial farms have severe negative impact on the earth. Wheat, corn, and soy from genetically modified seeds are grown to provide raw material for food manufacturers to process into "people" food, aka flour, sugar, and oil. The majority is provided to commercial farm feedlots. Monoculture crop farming uses chemical fertilizer, pesticides, and herbicides along with massive amount of water. These chemicals deplete the minerals and nutrients of the topsoil and wreck the environment with chemical runoff that drains into our waterways. Herbicides and pesticides are not effective when the weeds and pests become chemical resistant, so more chemicals are needed. This practice has decimated the living organisms in soil that plants need to thrive. Our land suffers when it is used for growing unhealthy grains for commercial feedlot of animals. Depleted topsoil will take time to recover from the toxic effects of chemicals. We need to support regenerative farming, crop rotation, and less chemical use, so we can turn dirt back into living soil for future generations.

The government subsidy of grains was supposed to help farmers and keep food cost stable and low. Currently, grain subsidies have mostly benefited commercial agricultural corporations and companies that produce and sell GMO seeds, pesticides, herbicides, fertilizers, and farming equipment. This situation has created cheap raw materials for the food manufacturers and for feedlots farms. For example, corn is used to feed animals in factory farms, made into HFCS, and ethanol. Less than ten percent of corn produced, is for human consumption. Soybeans are grown to provide cheap processed protein for animal feed and cheap soybean oil for processed foods. Cows that should be eating grass in pastures are fed processed grains, antacids, antibiotics, and growth hormones in factories. This type of farming is not good for them or for us. When our food source is full of processed grains, pesticides, antibiotics, or growth hormones, we suffer. We are being fed cheap, chemical-laced refined grains and poorly treated animals for corporate profit, not our health. The sooner we realize that, the sooner we can use our purchasing power to be heard and help make changes to our current food system, which sadly is not sustainable.

Variety is important. Many of us get bored if we eat the same foods over and over. Eating a variety of whole foods (raw, fermented, and cooked) will help build a good mix of microbial diversity in our guts and help us obtain needed nutrients. This collection of symbiotic microbes, which consist mostly of bacteria, thrives on whole foods with fiber. These microbes are hurt by repetitive use of antibiotics and many other drugs. Science has identified many strains that are associated with good and poor health. When we eat, we are not only feeding our bodies, we are populating our guts with probiotics, or microorganisms. They help keep our bodies healthy by production of needed substances such as vitamins, neurotransmitters, and enzymes. Having a healthy microbiome is crucial for health and longevity. The key is to have diversity to ensure balance. Not all microbes are all good or bad, but they are balanced to perform what they need to in order to survive and aid our survival. Having too much of a certain bacteria can be problematic and is common in modern diets, high in flour and sugar.

Fermented foods such as, sauerkraut, kimchi, pickles, miso, yogurt, and raw vegetables/fruits are great sources of probiotics. Taking quality probiotic supplements can be helpful in getting more strains of bacteria. It is important to note that having the multiple species of microorganisms is desirable; however, we need to feed them with natural prebiotics (soluble and insoluble fibers) found in plants, nuts, and seeds, so that they will thrive. Here is where most of our immunity resides and mental health is affected. Our brain and intestines (guts) are linked by constant communications, and a positive effect on one will positively affect the other. For example, serotonin, an important neurotransmitter, is largely produced in the gut and is used for brain cell communications.

Having a diet rich in sugar will lead to more growth of a certain type of gut bacteria that dominate your intestines. Just like how eating lots of candy with sugar can feed the bacteria in your mouth, resulting in cavities and gum disease. Changing the composition of your gut microbiome will take time. It is the cumulative effect of what you have been eating your whole life.

Understanding what our bodies need or do not need is a first step. It will be difficult foe some people to reduce the amount of sugar and processed foods in their diet, but this is temporary. There is joy to be discovered in eating whole real foods with healthy fats. Our taste buds will recalibrate when not exposed to sugar frequently. Finding replacements for or reducing processed foods is not easy because it is what we have been eating for the past fifty years.

Having been told that grains, in the form of bread, pasta, cereal, or crackers, are good for us is a misinformation mistake of the dated government guidelines of the US Department of Agriculture or USDA's food pyramid introduced in 1992. Grains and grain products were at the bottom of the pyramid, showing us that we are to eat more of it. The USDA revised their advice from the pyramid model to the MyPlate model in 2011, making vegetables and fruit a bigger part of the meal. Most people are unaware of this update. Although an improvement, it is still advocating grains, whole grains, and placing dairy as a food group separate from protein, which is unnecessary since dairy is not required by the body and should be optional. Although whole grain is better than refined grain, whole grain, when refined, as whole grain flour is not much better than white flour. It is used in many processed foods including bread and cereal. The guidelines were flawed from the beginning and are still flawed today.

The low fat and low cholesterol dietary advice based on historical science to promote heart health contributed to more grain and sugar consumption. To avoid fat, many turn to bread and pasta for the bulk of their diet. This resulted in excess energy with high glucose and high insulin response in the blood. When subjected to this cycle of glucose spikes multiple times daily for years, the population suffers. It is not what our bodies were designed to handle. Many people still think that sugar and flour are better options to eat than fat, based on these dated guidelines. The truth is that we need to raise our HDL (high-density lipoprotein) cholesterol levels to promote heart and brain health. We can do this by ignoring these dated guidelines and eat more natural fats and avoid sugar.

Butter and animal fats were replaced with margarine and vegetable oils in an attempt to improve heart health. The fear of saturated fats have driven the food industry to find creative ways of making food with "healthier" fats. They found that artificially saturating vegetable oils with hydrogen can achieve the taste and feel of nature made fat, with long shelf life. This partially hydrogenated oil became widely used in homes and in food factories. Another name for this product is trans fat, which have been found to cause inflammation and contribute to heart disease. The FDA (U. S. Food and Drug Administration), in 2015, started banning the use of trans fat in food based on overwhelming data of its ill effects. The manufacturers were given a grace period to comply. Currently, there are still many packaged foods like pies, cookies, peanut butter, and bread, made with trans fats on store shelves.

Whole foods, such as, nuts, seeds, seafood, and meat, coconut, have combinations of natural saturated and unsaturated fats. Our bodies can readily use natural fats in any form. We just don't have the enzymes to metabolize trans fats. We should be thinking in terms of nature made or factory-made fats. The former has been in our food supplies for thousands of years, and the latter from the modern industrial age.

The fat found in nature may or may not be saturated and is usually found in combination and is intended for human consumption as in coconut oil, olive oil, or animal fat. It is required for raw material for cell membranes and as fuel for energy, along with providing satiety signals, so we stop eating when we have had enough. Low fat food on the other hand does not satisfy and make us eat more than we need to. There is confusing nutritional advice about poly-saturated, mono-saturated, poly-unsaturated, and mono-unsaturated fats/oils. We don't need to analyze or know all about the components of fat and oils to enjoy the benefits of nature provided foods. Thinking that fat makes us fat, that natural saturated fat gives you heart disease, and that vegetable oil, refined from grains or seeds like cotton seed, soybeans, or corn, is heart healthy, is some of the wrong information we need to get right. Just keep in mind that food close to its original form is recognizable to our bodies, while factory made food can be harmful.

The invention and manufacturing of high fructose corn syrup (HFCS) is the latest insult to our health. HFCS is made from cornstarch. It is cheaper and sweeter than sugar. Since HFCS replaced sugar in sodas and many processed foods in the last few decades, it was blamed as a major cause of the obesity epidemic. Like refined sugar, when consumed in high frequency and amount, it can cause metabolic disorders like insulin resistance, type 2 diabetes, and fatty liver disease. With higher fructose content, the adverse effect of this liquid "sugar" is accelerated. Nutrition and dietary advice still tell us to eat fewer calories, lean protein, more whole grain, reduce saturated fats, and move more. The healthcare industry is still stuck in a count your calories mode, so sugar and fructose are free to wreck our bodies. Where are the harsh criticisms of sugar, HFCS, and processed foods in our food supply? Food corporations advocating 'eat fewer calories and move more' is often heard and believed. They also promote personal freedom and responsibility, which means that it is your own fault if you get sick from eating too much and exercising too little. They deflect their responsibility in the health crisis, because a calorie is a calorie. They are not interested in anyone's health but the health of their profits. All calories are not equal. Sugar, HFCS, and alcohol have calories; however, they are not real food. They can be enjoyed occasionally, but over consumption is far too common.

Changes in our thinking about food and our eating behaviors need to happen to maintain health. There are two major ingredients (flour and sugar) that we need to reduce or eliminate. In theory, this should be easy, but it is not. It has been ingrained in our lives as every day food and celebratory food. Our addiction to easily digestible carbs is hard to overcome. Eating tasty vegetables cooked with healthy fats and spices along with well-seasoned proteins that provide long-term satiety can help us get off the carb cravings and hunger cycles. When we no longer rely on refined carbs for fuel, we can enjoy it periodically or in smaller portions. Being flexible and diverse is good for our bodies. It is the weaning off part that is hard to do.

Not all carbohydrates are equal. Carbs from whole plants have nutrients, and fiber, while refined carbs are sugar and flour. They lack fiber and nutrients. The term "low carbs" or "high carbs" are meaningless; they are relative and do not define what kind of carbs they are and whether they are refined or whole plant. There is a big difference.

There is a common misunderstanding that eating plant based is healthy and good for the earth. Plant-based foods do not always mean healthy foods. It is the degree of processing. For example, sodas, candies, breads, cereals, and donuts can all be plant-based foods. These are highly processed, not good for frequent consumption, and not good for the planet. Substituting meat with processed GMO soybean (tofu), corn, or processed grain products with questionable chemicals does not make it good for your body or the environment. The ingredients should be scrutinized to determine degree of health or environmental benefits. Plant based can be healthy if the plants are whole and minimally processed.

Here are a few recommendations for eco-friendly food choices:

- Aim for a few varied and colorful, non-starchy vegetables like peppers, lettuce, broccoli, asparagus, spinach, cucumber, kale, or zucchini per day.
- Choose organic, seasonal, local, whole food products whenever possible.
- Choose pasture raised, free-range, antibiotic/hormone-free animal products, and eggs, whenever possible.
- When looking at packaged foods, choose the least processed options available with short ingredient list, natural/recognizable ingredients, minimal preservatives, and additives.

2. Sugar and Fructose

The word sugar can be confusing since it typically means glucose, fructose, or the combination of both. In nature, as in honey, fruits and vegetables, both glucose and fructose are combined, along with fiber, minerals, and vitamins. Fruits and vegetables provide us with needed nutrients like potassium, magnesium, and vitamins. Their availability is limited to seasons and like any fresh foods, has limited shelf life.

Table sugar or sucrose is considered to be a natural product by some. It is in fact a processed food very different from the source it came from. It is sometimes referred to as pure granulated sugar. "Pure" in this case means it is purely refined and processed to remove all traces of nutrient or fiber.

Hundreds of years ago, creative and persistent humans were able to extract the sweetness from sugarcanes. This extraction resulted in concentrated sweet liquid that eventually became granulated crystals. These crystals can be stored, transported, and sold to people all over the world. An industry was formed to mass-produce and distribute this highly coveted substance with the name table sugar, granulated sugar, or just sugar.

Historically, this sugar product was expensive due to the cost involved in manufacturing, transportation, and distribution. Only the wealthy could afford to buy it. Type 2 diabetes was still a rare condition and was only prevalent amongst the wealthier population. It was considered to be a disease of the rich.

Today, sugar is not expensive and available to all industrialized nations. The invention of sodas and processed foods has dramatically increased the consumption of sugar all over the world. The ill effects that followed did not occur right away. It took decades. We currently have an epidemic of metabolic diseases, which is likely the result of the cumulative frequent sugar consumption.

Chemically, sugar or sucrose is a simple carbohydrate with one glucose molecule and one fructose molecule bound together. When ingested, the body will break the bond of the two molecules. The glucose is easily absorbed and used by the whole body for energy. The fructose is carried to the liver to be metabolized. This is where the damage occurs. The frequency, speed, and amount that the liver processes fructose dictates its health. When there is excessive fructose, more than the liver can handle, it is stored as fat in the liver. Overtime, too much accumulated fat, will damage the organ and impair its many functions.

Glucose provides us with energy in the form of adenosine triphosphate, or ATP with a byproduct of carbon dioxide. Fructose depletes the body of ATP when it is metabolized in the liver. When ATP is consumed instead of being produced, this can signal the body into fat conservation mode. The book *Nature Wants Us to Be Fat* by Richard J. Johnson, MD, explains how this survival mechanism works. This signaling is a survival mechanism where fat is stored in the body to help it survive famine or hibernation in the case of wild animals before winter. Frequent, high-volume consumption of fructose can manifest itself as insulin resistance, type 2 diabetes, fatty liver, and may lead to cirrhosis of the liver. The effect is the same as over-consumption of alcohol. Alcohol, or ethanol is fermented sugar. Both sugar and alcohol affect the liver in the same way. The effect of high fructose consumption was not designed to hurt you but to save you from possible famine by generating body fat. Historically, humans don't have constant access to food, famine or dry spell is common and those with body fat will be able to survive until food is found. This fasting period allows the body to use up fat stored in the liver and on the body. Our modern-day diet, with high amount of fructose, can impair the liver and hijack the fat regulation of the body and inadvertently harm us because we never have to go without food and never need to access stored fat for survival.

Recent research confirmed more negative effects of fructose as detailed in *Drop Acid* by David Perlmutter, MD. In metabolizing fructose, the body produces uric acid. High uric acid levels have been associated with a prevalence of gout, a painful joint condition. It has been demonstrated that high uric acid levels result in high blood pressure, insulin resistance, and many other chronic metabolic conditions. Uric acid is also produced in response to many activities such as exercising or fasting, but it is temporary and is excreted out of the body through the kidneys. When insulin level is high (in people with insulin resistance or type 2 diabetes), sodium and uric acid does not get excreted properly. This can lead to a vicious cycle resulting in continually high uric acid levels that leads to metabolic disorders.

Another effect of fructose has been linked to mental hyperactivity. In nature, animals need to forage for food to eat and store fat for the winter. Initiated by eating a lot of ripe fruit, high in fructose, they develop a risk-taking, impulsive personality with characteristics of attention deficit and hyperactivity disorder (ADHD). High fructose consumption has been shown to affect mental activities of animals and is linked to hyperactivity and impulsiveness in people, especially children.

Fructose does not promote satiety. Instead, it increases thirst and appetite, which can lead to ingesting of more fructose. Fructose is also responsible for creating another condition that makes us overeat. It makes us less sensitive to the leptin hormone. This hormone is needed to help provide satiety signals to our brain.

Juice, initially seen as healthy, since it is from fruit and may have vitamins and minerals, may not be good for us depending on the amount being consumed. It is mostly fructose but devoid of actual fruit which has fibers and other micronutrients. It is the fiber that prevents the fructose from going right to the liver by slowing down the absorption and letting the body digest slowly as nature intended. Imagine eating ten oranges, which is hard to do, as opposed to drinking a glass of orange juice. The effect of fructose from juice may be worse than a sugared drink, since it is mostly fructose.

The sugar industry, corn refiners industry, and food/drink corporations have made sugar and HFCS easily available, so everyone can consume more of it. To say sugar is healthier than HFCS is to say jumping off a ten-story building is better than jumping off an eleven-story building. HFCS does have a unique characteristics not found in sugar. The higher fructose content is one (55% to 65%), another one is that there is no bond between the fructose and glucose molecule. Once ingested, they don't need to be separated by our bodies so the time to be metabolized is more rapid and so is the negative effect. They are both damaging to the body and dependent on the amount and frequency of consumption. They are not essential for survival and are harmful in excess.

The following are general guidelines for sugar consumption from the American Heart Association (AHA) and the US Department of Agriculture (USDA). This advice should be for healthy individuals. If you are suffering from any metabolic disease (over one third of the population), the amount should be lower. This information is not known by most people and is likely to stay that way if food corporations want to sell more products and healthcare does not prioritize the importance of food.

Below are sugar limit recommendations from the AHA and USDA.

The American Heart Association (AHA) [1]

Daily sugar limit recommendations for men and women.

Men should consume no more than 9 teaspoons (36 grams or 150 calories) of added sugar per day.

For women, the number is lower, that is, 6 teaspoons (25 grams or 100 calories) per day.

USDA Guidelines from **The Dietary Guidelines for Americans, 2020-2025**, Executive Summary[2]

Added sugars—Less than 10 percent of calories per day starting at age 2. Avoid foods and beverages with added sugars for those younger than age 2.

The AHA's advice above is more precise than the USDA's advice, which is based on percentages. The USDA Dietary Guidelines say that adults should get no more than 10 percent of total calories from added sugars. This information is vague and not helpful in deciding how much is too much. Not many people will do the math. Assuming 1 teaspoon of sugar equals 15 calories, if a person takes in 2000 calories a day, which means 200 calories can come from sugar, and that equates to 13 teaspoons or 52 g. This is higher than the AHA's Guidelines. Many people consume more than both the AHA's and USDA's recommendations every day. A 12-ounce can of soda with 39 g of sugar exceed the AHA's recommended daily limit for women.

The USDA recommends that those less than two years old abstain or avoid added sugars. This information is important but is not well known, and neither are the adult recommendations. Everyday foods contain sugars and HFCS that we may not be aware of, for example, bread, soup, sauces, ketchup, and crackers. A slice of bread can have up to 4g of added sugar. A small yogurt cup or can of soup may have more sugar than a can of soda. Paying attention to labels will help us see how much sugar was added. Since sugar is added to most processed foods, eating whole foods will give us more control over how much sugar is consumed.

Excessive intake of sugars and HFCS causes high blood pressure, heart disease, chronic inflammation, fatty liver disease, and type 2 diabetes.[3] Sugar will not kill you right away, but in the long term, excessive exposure will wear down your body. To some, it is sooner, especially children who start consuming sugar early and often. Drinking sugared beverages, including smoothies, can overwhelm your body with an excessive amount of sugar. Nature never intended for us to metabolize so much and so frequently. The body can handle it because it is trying to help you survive, but year after year, it can be damaged if we don't change our eating or drinking habits. We should not wait for stricter advice from healthcare professionals. Many may still be convinced that fat and calories are to blame.

Sugar consumption has drastically increased all over the world, and people are not aware of how toxic the effects are until they are diagnosed with some type of metabolic disease. Even when diagnosed with pre-diabetes or metabolic diseases like type 2 diabetes or fatty liver, people are not told to stop consuming sugar. These conditions are blamed on luck, genes, overeating, or lack of exercise. Our genetics or physical activities may play a role in fending off the disease, but long term, our food choices affect us.

Understanding what is happening in our environment is crucial to making changes for the better. Our health and quality of life is under our control if we know what to start eliminating. There are many who advocate the elimination or major reduction of sugar in our diets. Their voices are diluted by many mixed messages pointing to other causes like too much salt, fat, calories, and lack of exercise. Sugar and HFCS are not the only toxins out there, but the need to reduce them is important for our long-term health.

Some common names for processed sugar found on food labels:

brown sugar   corn sweetener
corn syrup   fruit juice concentrates
high-fructose corn syrup   honey
invert sugar   malt sugar
molasses   syrup

Look for sugar molecules ending in "ose" (dextrose, fructose, glucose, lactose, maltose, sucrose).

Dr. Daryl Gioffre sums it up well here:

With an average American consuming 38 teaspoons of sugar a day, it's putting ourselves and our kids on a sugar and stress-eating rollercoaster!

This is a worrying fact because our bodies can only metabolize 6 teaspoons a day! So, anything after that becomes a poison and neurotoxin to our body.

For helpful information and guide on how to become less addicted to sugar, the book by Dr. Daryl Gioffre, *Get off Your Sugar* may be helpful.

3. Refined Grains (Flour) and Wheat

Flour, especially wheat flour, is associated with comfort food. It is the main ingredient of breads, bagels, pastas, crackers, cakes, pies, and pizzas. It is inexpensive and stores for months or years, without going bad. It has been part of our civilization for thousands of years. It has helped us survive famines, natural disasters, winters, and wars.

Recently we are hearing more about negative effects of wheat and gluten. In moderate amount, it is not harmful to most of us. The amount we consume recently has increased substantially, enough to provide us with adverse effects. By becoming the largest part of our diet, it has crowded out whole foods, especially vegetables, proteins, and fats. Flour, a refined grain is easily incorporated into processed, packaged foods can be found everywhere and is usually eaten at every meal. Although it may be enriched with vitamins to help make it better for us, it is not the ideal food choice. Flour is a processed food that lacks nutrients and is full of energy dense simple carbohydrates. Eating too much provides us with excess glucose that requires insulin to process. Our bodies are design to hoard glucose and store it for future use in cases of famine.

Whole-wheat flour may be advertised as better for us because it has more fiber. That may be true, but it is a processed food with added processed fibers, not really whole grain. The whole grain was pulverized to make whole-grain flour and affects the body the same way flour does. Fiber from whole foods, has both soluble and insoluble fiber. It is needed in our intestines to help regulate the absorption of glucose and nutrients, along with feeding our symbiotic microbes in our guts.

Modern wheat, corn, and soybeans, grown on commercial farms, have only existed in the past fifty plus years. Their seeds have been genetically modified to tolerate more herbicides, and pesticides. Eating these grains will introduce these chemicals in to our bodies. Chemicals like glyphosate (Round-up) will adversely affect our gut health by killing off microorganisms, which are part of a healthy body. In addition, the liver will have to work harder to remove the chemical toxins, making it less efficient in performing other functions. Because processed grains are so fine, it easily converts to glucose and goes directly into our blood stream and raises our blood glucose level quickly. The human digestive system was designed to process whole foods, not factory made and easily digestible foods. It has been the last fifty years that we have been eating this highly refined modern wheat in huge amounts. Some of us cannot tolerate this product. Since it is a major food source for most, it is a possible cause of many common health ailments.

Commercial wheat is modified to have quick harvest and higher yield. Typically, wheat is mostly carbohydrates and about 10–15 percent protein. Of all the total protein, 80 percent is gluten. Modern wheat has higher gluten content and many more proteins as a result of crossbreeding and genetic modifications. These created proteins have never been seen or digested by humans before and was never tested for safe human consumption. We are the guinea pigs of this modern wheat project. Due to similar chemical structures to endorphins, some proteins are considered to be exorphins, binding to our opiate brain cell receptors, making us feel good and wanting more. This wheat is also being associated with autoimmune diseases, arthritis, hair loss, and mental health issues. Many suffer from food allergies, or unexplained body inflammation, which can be eliminated sometimes by taking the wheat out of the diet. The book *Wheat Belly* by William Davis, MD, is recommended reading for those wanting to explore wheat's ill effects on the body.

To minimize adverse effects, make refined grains, flour (pasta, bread) organic when possible and a smaller part of your meal. All necessary macronutrients and micronutrients can come from other whole foods like meat, seafood, nuts, seeds, fruits, or vegetables. Refined grain is not a necessary part of the diet. Whole grains are historically a food source that helped humanity survive when no other foods were available; it is no longer the same grain and not essential for survival. We no longer have a survival issue but an overabundance of flour and processed foods.

There are many whole grains available today that are not refined and can be part of our diet, depending on preferences, such as oats, buckwheat, rice, or quinoa.

In addition to exposure to toxins, promoting addiction to flour, and elevating blood glucose levels, there is another negative effect of frequent consumption of refined grains. Flour, when digested, primarily becomes glucose, an energy source in the body. In excess, it can contribute to "advanced glycation end products" or AGE. This is a natural process in the body where excess glucose binds with various proteins to create a useless product that may disrupt parts of the body, like cataracts in the eye or atherosclerosis in blood vessels, or in the brain resulting in cognitive decline. The key here is excess. Our bodies have to keep up with the glucose load we ingest, and if we take in too much, the excess will result in AGE. These conditions are associated with aging and are accelerated in people with poor glucose control, like those with diabetes. To look at it another way, to slow the aging process and deterioration of the body, we should maintain optimal glucose levels, and keep it steady to prevent premature aging. Eating foods that minimizes the fluctuation of glucose is a simple first step. Whole foods, plant or animal based, with natural fats, protein, and lots of fiber, will not put your glucose level on a roller coaster ride like refined grains do.

About Gluten:

Gluten, a protein in some grains, mostly wheat, is one major source of inflammation for those sensitive to it. Celiac disease is a condition where the gut cannot tolerate the gluten protein. This sensitivity to gluten can affect the gut and now has been shown to affect the brain or body of many people, resulting in chronic inflammation. Testing negative for celiac disease does not mean you are not sensitive to gluten or some other protein in wheat. Many people have been able to alleviate unwanted symptoms when wheat and gluten are eliminated. Even if you are not sensitive, eating less is better, especially if it is replaced by natural whole foods.

4. Fats and Oils (Good and Bad)

What determines if a certain fat or oil is good for us? Where it comes from, and how much it is processed. Minimally processed natural fats and oils include, coconut oil, butter, cold pressed or extra virgin olive oil, lard, fatty fish, and fatty meat. All these fats are composed of saturated and unsaturated fatty acids. In nature, they exist together in different proportions. We were not meant to dissect it apart and try to eat only one kind or another. All are vital and have numerous health benefits. Ancient humans would eat nutritious fatty organ meat first and leave muscle meat last since it is less nutritious.

The word "saturated" has been demonized because it means that the oil can harden at room temperature and has been mistakenly linked to heart disease. It is not the natural saturated fats that cause heart disease; it is the artificially saturated oils, or partially hydrogenated oils, known as trans fats that are harmful.

Industrial oils, trans fats, partially or fully hydrogenated oils, vegetable oil, corn oil, canola oil, soybean oil, cottonseed oil, Crisco, and margarine should be avoided. They are highly processed and are common food additives providing processed foods with a long shelf life. Trans fats are firmly linked to inflammation, heart disease, and vascular disease. Trans fats have been banned but can still be found as an ingredient in many processed foods. Vegetable oils have not been banned but have damaged us by being sold to the public as heart-healthy oil since they are from a vegetable and have no cholesterol. It is high in omega 6 fatty acids, which when not balanced by omega 3 fatty acids, is linked to inflammation and poor health when consumed in large amounts. It is not heart healthy as advertised. It is mostly refined from commercially grown soybean or corn.

In 1794, the cotton industry was able to produce and export large amounts of cotton fibers after the invention of the cotton gin. The seeds of the cotton plants were the only things that remained. They were useless, until the process of refining was invented several years later, through mechanical and chemical means at high temperatures. From the seeds, oil was produced. At that time, it was able to make up for a dwindling supply of whale oil. Cottonseed oil was produced and sold for industrial applications. Although cotton is not food, somehow cottonseed oil became sold as a food product. To stabilize the oil from going rancid quickly and mimic natural fat, the process of hydrogenation (adding hydrogen to the oil) was discovered. The product became Crisco (crystallized cotton seed oil) in the year 1911. This process hardens the oil at room temperature and mimics natural fats like lard and butter at a much cheaper price. This product made baked and fried foods taste good but was never tested on humans for harmful effects.

Humans did not evolve to digest artificial trans fats. We lack the enzymes to break it down, and the fat cannot be used for energy or cannot be removed properly by our digestive system, so inflammation throughout the body may occur, which can lead to hardening or compromised endothelial vessels and heart disease. It is also been shown to raise the bad LDL cholesterol in the blood. The FDA started banning of the product in 2015, but has extended the grace period many times.

Our bodies need natural fat and cholesterol to function properly. It is required for many things, including production of hormones, cell membranes and myelin sheath for nerve cells. It is vital for the absorption of fat-soluble vitamins. Not having enough healthy fats can lead to sub-optimal health. Consuming fat does not affect our blood glucose level.

Insulin is not required or released in this process unlike the consumption of carbohydrates, which breaks down to glucose, resulting in insulin production.

Many are afraid of fat because of two unfortunate things. They were told to avoid fat to prevent heart disease and to eat fewer calories to not gain weight. As it turned out, we need healthy fat for our hearts and brains. Our body weight is not always dependent on calories.

Natural fats like in butter, eggs, cheese, coconut oil, avocado, lard, olive oil, seafood, and fatty meat can be enjoyed as part of a varied and balanced diet. They are needed to provide fatty acids, cholesterol, and satiety. Processed, low or no-fat products like yogurt, milk, cheese, or ultra-processed foods are not helping anyone lose weight or become healthy. Fat is not the problem, but a lack of natural fat can be.

5. Salt

Salt (sodium chloride) can be a controversial subject. Many have claimed that too much causes hypertension (high blood pressure) and heart disease. Based on information from the book *The Salt Fix* by Dr. James Dinicolantonio, I think we can all use another perspective on the subject. This claim is another past recommendation based on flimsy science that has permeated our thinking and that of our healthcare providers. The message to reduce salt does not always help and may even hurt those with heart conditions that need sodium for proper cellular signaling.

We can all agree on the fact that we would not be alive if our bodies did not have necessary electrolytes, one being sodium. Along with calcium, potassium, and magnesium, these minerals long with many other, are vital for proper functioning of the body. Our blood, soft tissues, and bones store these essential minerals. A healthy individual without any kidney or metabolic issues can excrete excess salt through sweat and urine. It is easier for the body to excrete excess salt than to recapture and recycle salt when it does not have enough. With this vital nutrient, there is an optimal dose that the body needs, and we have in inherent physical signaling such as, taste buds that allow us to determine if something is salty, when we are thirsty, or when we have cravings for salty foods. This has kept us alive for thousands of years. It is one of our survival instincts.

This "check and balance" system can become compromised when we consume salt with sugar. Sugar has no feedback feature to tell us we have had enough; in fact, it makes us want more, so we consume more of both salt and sugar. Consuming more water will reduce the concentration of salt in our bodies but will not change the amount of fructose delivered to the liver. Excess salt can be excreted, but the body stores excess sugar. Most people are not hurting for salt if they eat regularly. If you are sweating for an extended amount of time or if you are fasting, you may have to supplement with electrolytes that includes salt. This is true for sweating athletes, especially in the summer when muscle cramps are common due to lost of minerals.

Salt does not cause hypertension, but the reduction of salt will slightly lower blood pressure. This is a small Band-Aid fix. The most common cause of hypertension, sugar and refined grains in the diet, have not been properly identified and therefore have not been removed. The advice to reduce salt is still being given. It is better to identify and correct the true causes of hypertension and not be distracted by the stubborn common "wisdom" of eating less salt.

Consumption of sugar provides both carbohydrate and fructose to the body. Excess amount of glucose will be stored as glycogen in the liver and muscle. The metabolism of fructose, which happens mostly in the liver, results in production of uric acid. More fructose results in more uric acid in the body. The latest science has demonstrated the connection between prolonged high uric acid levels and hypertension, decreased nitric oxide in the blood, brain, and heart, resulting in insulin resistance. The book *Drop Acid* by David Perlmutter, MD, provides details about uric acid and how it can negatively affect our bodies. This information is recent and should be included in the discussion regarding hypertension for the general population.

Being dehydrated for an extended amount of time can trigger a survival mechanism. We may start to store fat for possible future famine when we lack water. Richard J. Johnson, MD, explores this subject in his book, *Nature Wants Us to Be Fat*. He explained how animals and people gain weight by triggering a survival "switch" to store fat as a result of many things like excessive fruit(fructose) consumption and dehydration. In famine, fat is metabolized for energy and as a byproduct, provides water to the body. To prevent this fat production mechanism from occurring, adequate hydration or drinking more water is recommended.

Salt regulation can be impaired by many conditions. For example, having a chronically high insulin level will prevent the kidneys from adequately excreting salt. Due to a large percentage of the population suffering from insulin resistance and kidney disease, there are more people with compromised salt regulation and kidney issues. These and many other conditions are valid reasons to limit salt intake. Although it may be necessary, limiting salt is not a cure for the actual problem. Finding the true cause of the problem and healing what needs to be healed should be the goal.

Our ancestors ate much more salt than we do. They salted and fermented foods to keep them from spoiling since they did not have refrigeration. They did not suffer from chronic metabolic diseases, eating and excreting salt was not a problem.

I believe that salt was guilty by association when it was actually sugar that is damaging. Salt is necessary for our survival, whereas sugar is not and can be harmful if not limited. Unrefined salt is recommended since it is not processed and, therefore, contains trace minerals our bodies need.

Iodine, thyroid health, and salt[4]:

In 1924, in an effort to improve public health, the U. S. Food and Drug Administration (FDA) urged salt makers to add iodine to salt and then urged the population to use salt liberally. They even gave "goiter pills," which are large doses of iodine, to children in school. This was successful in eliminating goiters (enlarged thyroid glands), some mental and physical impairment in people, especially children. This condition was more common to people living inland or in rural areas where seafood or sea vegetables were not available. Iodine is a necessary nutrient for the thyroid gland to work properly. Without proper functioning thyroid, hormone levels are inadequate which may result in growth and metabolism impairment in children and adults. Goiter is a condition when thyroid glands struggle to get iodine so it becomes enlarged trying to capture iodine from the body. Iodized salt and potassium iodine (KI) are prescribed to reverse goiter, thyroid problems, and other health conditions.

After the 1960s, in response to reports that salt causes heart disease and hypertension, the general wisdom forgot about goiter and iodine, and urged people to cut back on salt. Currently, the reduction of salt has not reduced heart disease or improved health in the population since the advice was given, as shown by the growing numbers of people with heart conditions, metabolic abnormalities, autoimmune disease, and thyroid issues.

Today the salt in our diets may lack the required iodine and other minerals if we are eating more processed and fast foods than cooking meals. Cooking with iodized salt, eating seafood, or sea vegetables, will provide more iodine for optimal thyroid health. Supplements in the form of potassium iodine or multiple vitamins with iodine can help ensure that we have adequate amount. Not having goiter does not mean your iodine level is optimal. If you have health issues, knowing if you are iodine deficient is something that can be easily corrected.

Some symptoms of severe iodine deficiency:

Goiters (enlarged thyroid glands)
Impaired growth and learning in children
Increased risk for heart attacks and failures
Lack of thyroid hormones – slow death

6. Eat-Fast Balance

Eating and drinking is vital for life. It is the way we take in energy and nutrients to stay alive. Hunting, fishing, gathering, and farming are activities that we used to perform to get the needed food materials. This process takes time and does not produce food consistently. From one day to the next ancient people really don't know when they will eat. Their bodies, like ours, were designed to tolerate periods of food and lack of food. The balance kept them lean and strong. Fast forward to our modern era, food is always available. We no longer have to wait for the harvest or hunt to eat. What and when we eat is determined by us now, not nature.

What has changed the last few decades is the idea that snacks are required to keep us from overeating at meals, keep our blood sugar stable, and to keep our metabolism from slowing down. Was this scientific findings or marketing slogans? It is not a stretch to assume that marketers will use any hint of science in their slogans to sell products. They want us to eat more food and snacks more often so they can profit. The norm has changed. We are encouraged to snack, have dessert every day, and even eat while driving. The "forced" fasting created by nature has disappeared. The only time we practice fasting is during sleep. This practice is vital and needed now more than ever. We need to know that we can go for several hours or even days without food.

Low blood sugar is not a problem if you are healthy. Your body's survival mechanism requires that your blood glucose level be automatically regulated, like your heart rate. You can still function. In fact, if you are healthy, your brain is more alert when you are hungry. Your body was designed to hunt and find food. It's a survival instinct.

We have been led to believe that eating constantly is healthy. This is not true. Snacking all day does not make you speed up your metabolism. Eating stimulates your appetite, like an appetizer before a meal and induces insulin production, which puts our bodies/cells into growth and energy storage mode. Being in the feeding state constantly can throw our hormones out of balance. These are hormones that interact and dictate our metabolism and fat regulations.

Eating frequently is taxing on your digestive system. The pancreas, which produces enzymes to breakdown food and insulin to help carry glucose into cells, should not be working all the time. We are more like lions (hunt when hungry) than cows (grazes in pasture all day) when it comes to ideal eating habits. Our bodies are designed to endure feast and famine. It was never designed to feast all the time. Time and calorie restricted experiments on animals show longevity with less frequent feedings, even if the total amount of food was kept the same.

There are many benefits to fasting on the body and on the cellular level. When food is available, cells focus on growth and when food is not available, the focus is on elimination and repair. The body produces human growth hormones (HGH) and brain-derived neurotropic factors (BDNF) when in the fasting state. These proteins are vital for metabolic health and brain health (learning and memory). Intermittent fasting triggers regeneration of new cells including immune system cells, which not only boosts our immunity but also plays a role in longevity.

Another reason people may want to eat constantly is that food has become a coping mechanism for boredom, stress, or unhappiness. The joy of eating food is real and has helped our species survive. When eating becomes an obsession, it may be because it can be mentally and physically addictive, especially when high in sugar or wheat content. Sugar and wheat are addictive to most people at varying degrees. There is no easy way to get off the sugar and carb addiction. Being aware and educated is a good place to start if you have this struggle.

Fasting is not recommended for people with any form of eating disorder. It is also not usually recommended for children or pregnant women.

There is no set amount of times that you have to eat per day. Breakfast, lunch, and dinner are social, convenient, practices. Our bodies store excess food energy as glycogen and fat for future use. We naturally hoard fat since we don't know when the next famine is coming. Most of us never see famine, so we always have liver and muscle full of glycogen. When glycogen store is low, as a result of not eating for many hours or extensive exercise, we can use ketones for the majority of our fuel needs by metabolizing fat, which is an energy source that is more efficient than glucose and can meet the body's energy needs easily. Being able to use ketones when glucose is low is ideal. To optimize our bodies, we should work with what nature has provided, a flexible and efficient body.

Some of us are not able to switch fuel sources easily if we always rely on glucose for fuel and never need to access fat stores. There may be uncomfortable physical symptoms for those trying to fast or eat less carbohydrate. This may be referred to as keto-flu or carbohydrate addiction, which is the body rebelling against change or glucose withdrawal symptoms. Some symptoms include brain fog, fatigue, headaches, and chills. Fasting by slowly increasing fasting time and eating healthy fats and proteins may help. A state of ketosis is when the primary source of energy is ketones.

Many religions have incorporated fasting as part of their practice. It is a form of devotion, self-sacrifice, or extending food supply. For whatever other reasons, it is good for general health.

A major benefit to fasting is that our bodies will stay sensitive to insulin because our cells are not exposed to insulin continuously. Having less frequent exposure to insulin will help prevent insulin resistance and protect the pancreas. See *The Complete Guide to Fasting* by Dr. Jason Fung for helpful fasting advice and strategies. Some fasting strategies are flexible and can be easily incorporated into our lifestyle.

Intermittent fasting is now being considered for the treatment of type 2 diabetes[5]. Skipping meals or eating every other day can be forms of fasting. Benefits may include weight loss, but a better benefit is helping the body become sensitive to insulin and eventually reverse type 2 diabetes. This practice, along with eating less refined grains and sugar to maintain a stable glucose level, is effective and may not require medication. For many on medication, a reduction, and eventually an end to medication may be achieved. If you are on medication, it is important to check with your healthcare provider before changing your diet or fasting.

Eating is a pleasure that should be enjoyed leisurely at appropriate times. Eating less frequently can bring more pleasure to each meal and protect the health of our metabolic process. Fasting between meals is a good place to start.

Fasting and Hibernation:

Many wild animals, like bears and squirrels, rely on body fat for energy when they hibernate. They survive several winter months without eating by metabolizing their stored body fat while sleeping. They don't need to take in water since metabolizing fat results in a byproduct of water. They wake up to a smaller body with less fat and will eventually start to prepare for winter again by eating.

7. Sleep and Movement

Sleep is crucial for optimal health. A good quality sleep of seven to nine hours each night is recommended by most experts. During sleep, the brain and body go through many necessary steps in order to properly repair, detoxify, organize, and optimize their functions. Missing out on restorative sleep may impair your ability to think or function. Sleeping also gives us the opportunity to fast and give our digestive system a break. Just like eating is necessary and enjoyable, we should enjoy relaxation and sleep too.

For some, there is difficulty going to sleep or staying asleep. Modern day schedules may affect our natural circadian rhythm. This rhythm is set by our exposure to the sun. Our hormones are tied to the presence and absence of sunlight. It is advisable to expose your eyes to sunlight when awake and avoid blue light at night. Melatonin, a hormone that we produce at night, is required for optimal sleep and many other functions. Many sleeping disorders can be attributed to a lack of adequate melatonin or other vitamins or minerals. Screen time with blue light at night has been shown to disrupt the circadian rhythm and trick our brains into thinking it is daytime. Many electronic devices like cell phones have a blue light-blocking mode to help with this condition.

Lack of sun light exposure can affect the circadian rhythm and the production of vitamin D, which is a required hormone that is created by sunlight exposure on the skin. Lack of vitamin D has many negative effects including poor sleep quality. Supplementation is highly recommended.

Magnesium deficiency is also common if our diets are lacking in nuts, seeds, and green leafy vegetables. Magnesium helps with melatonin regulation and activates neurotransmitters that are responsible for calming the body and the mind.

Another common sleep issue is disrupted breathing or sleep apnea. Ideally, breathing should be mostly through our noses. This is the optimal way the air is supposed to flow. For some, mouth breathing during sleep is common, and this habit will result in lower quality sleep with more snoring and dry mouth. Figuring out the cause of sleep issues and rectifying them will benefit our health.

Naps are common in many cultures. If not excessive, it is a natural way to recharge and rest. Shutting down for a little while can reset our bodies, especially our hard-working optic nerves and brain.

Movement and exercise are vital in helping to get quality sleep, and their importance is often overlooked. Daily physical movement is necessary for health. Our muscles, including the heart, need to work to maintain strength. Our bodies are designed to move, walk or run, for survival. Keeping muscles strong provides us with balance, agility, and protects our joints. Active movement provides increased oxygen input to the lungs and a faster heart rate to circulate the blood. This is vital to our health and a key to longevity. Blood is the source of growth, repair, and healing. Walking each day is a good start. Adding strength training, stretching, or other sports/activities to our routines are all good options.

There are many other benefits to movement and exercise beyond blood and oxygen circulation. It is also the circulation of our lymphatic fluids and the production of neurotransmitter chemicals like endorphins, dopamine, and serotonin, which are valuable for mental health. Exercise boosts the immune system, strengthens not just the body and all its processes but also the mitochondrial function of our cells. It also increases the number of mitochondria, making it more efficient and increases the length of our telomeres, which are important for proper cell division and DNA replication. (Telomeres are protein structures found at the end of each chromosome to protect genes from degradation.)

Having optimal sleep and daily movement is crucial to health and has been undervalued. Both sleep and movement help maintain brain and body health, through the complex regeneration, inflammation reduction, and healing process. This is what we have in our health "tool box", simple activities to optimize our survival and promote longevity.

8. Brain Health

The common misconception about our brain is that we are born with a finite amount of cells or neurons, and loose them as we age. Latest science tells us that this is not true. Brain cells, like other cells in the body, die and regenerate. We can grow new neurons, and strengthen their connections, which enhance brain cell communications. This is called neuroplasticity. We can maintain and optimize our brains through what we eat, our thoughts, our movements, sleep, and avoidance of toxins.

We all want to maintain our cognitive ability because it is our quality of life. It is scary to think that we can lose our minds literally to Alzheimer's disease, the most common form of dementia. Latest science tells us that we can have cognitive decline ten to twenty years before the symptoms appear. Currently, there is no medical treatment or medication that will cure this disease once it is fully established. The good news is that early onset of this condition may be reversed. Better news is that we can take steps now to help prevent it from happening. We can mitigate our risk with lifestyle interventions.

It is not surprising to know that we have an increase in the number of people diagnosed with Alzheimer's in the aging population. Age is a major risk factor since it takes years for the condition to develop. Currently, metabolic diseases, type 2 diabetes, and dementia have been diagnosed in younger populations. Toddlers and teenagers now are at risk for type 2 diabetes, and middle-aged adults are diagnosed with dementia, whereas these conditions were more common in old age. It is not a stretch to blame our food environment, which has changed much in the past fifty years. Having type 2 diabetes is a major risk factor for being diagnosed with dementia. Blood quality and condition of insulin resistance affect brain health. If your health providers are not telling you, it is because they may not have been exposed to latest science. We have the ability to help prevent cognitive decline. Luck and genetics play a smaller role than previously thought. Having the genetic marker, ApoE4, does not mean you are destined to develop Alzheimer's or other forms of dementia. Not having the marker does not mean you are safe from cognitive decline or dementia. You can mitigate your risk by food choices and lifestyle with or without the genetic marker. The book *The End of Alzheimer's Program* by Dr. Dale Bredesen has valuable information about preventative protocols to implement.

There is a strong connection and communication between our guts and our brain. This area of study is active and in the near future will provide us with more helpful information about our bodies. The book *Brain Maker* by Dr. David Perlmutter has fascinating details about gut and brain health, and how they affect each other. Poor gut health has been associated with depression, anxiety, diabetes, and obesity. Poor gut health can be attributed to poor nutrition, less diverse microbiome, and diet high in sugar and flour. Optimizing gut health will benefit brain health along with the rest of the body.

Food affects the health and type of the microbes we have in our guts. Some unacknowledged allergies or sensitivities to certain foods may contribute to poor gut and brain health. Gluten is one protein that is not tolerated in the gut of people with celiac disease. It has been established that gluten can cause inflammation in the brain and body of people sensitive to it even if they don't have celiac disease. Sugar is another substance that can negatively affect both our brain and guts. Not having required fatty acids or adequate cholesterol from food can impair growth of brain cells. Cell membranes and nerve cells need fat for proper formation.

Conditions to avoid for brain health:

Insulin resistance – When your brain is not sensitive to insulin, the brain cannot use glucose for energy, and the neurons cannot function well, and they may die prematurely.

Type 2 diabetes – Having diabetes increases your risk factor for Alzheimer's disease or other forms of dementia.

Avoid antidepressant or unnecessary medications – These are not cures, but symptom management options that may impede healing and affect gut health. See Chapter 14.

Avoid overuse of antibiotics and pain medications – When used frequently, these medications can adversely affect our gut microbiome and liver.

High levels of toxins – Chemical toxins or toxins from infections can have severe negative effect on the brain.

Nutrient deficiencies

Lack of adequate sleep

Conditions for maximizing brain health:

- Eating a variety of whole foods, low in sugar and flour. (Vitamin D3 and Omega-3 oil with EPA and DHA supplements are highly recommended.)
- Move or exercise daily.
- Using your brain by reading writing, enjoying various hobbies, or learning new skills is beneficial. Being able to focus, learn, or solve problems will help

strengthen neuron connections. More connections are valuable in preserving brain functions. Having many neuron connections is vital for communication, for processing speed, and for rerouting of information paths when there is an unforeseen obstruction. Not using these connections for extended period of time may result in losing connections. The best way to retain them is by using them.

- Practice mindfulness or meditation. It has been scientifically proven to provide benefits. For some people, prayers and meditation in a formal (religious) or personal setting provide the needed peace. The act of meditation like focusing on your thoughts (for example, concentration on breathing) is both easy and hard. Since our mind continually wanders, it needs to be redirected. The ability to control or redirect our thoughts and emotions can be difficult for some, but can be strengthened with practice. Reading is a good example of an activity that requires prolonged focus that also provides new information and thought formation. Yoga and Tai Chi are good examples of activities for both body movement and mindfulness. An App like 'Headspace' can be helpful with guided meditation. It provides simple guidance and lessons that is tailored to the individual.

- Manage excessive stress. Many people suffer from stress as a reaction to perceived, rather than actual life threatening situation. Managing stress means to have some control over how your mind reacts to situations. Prolonged stress can be harmful due to the constant release of cortisol, a vital hormone that activates the sympathetic nervous system known as the "fight or flight" mode. High, constant cortisol level may lead to chronic inflammation. Activities, like meditation, exercise, or hobbies can reduce cortisol levels and increase other relaxing hormones like oxytocin.

- Nurturing positive relationships with family and friends.
- Having a positive attitude and compassion for self and others.
- Focusing on gratitude for what we have and have to offer, can help us find peace and optimize our mental health.

9. Heart Health

The heart, like other organs, will thrive and heal when given energy, nutrients from food, adequate sleep, and regular exercises. Like the rest of the body, it is affected by many factors, like hormones, excess glucose, toxins, and stress.

Heart medication and procedures have saved numerous lives and continue to extend the lives of patients with heart disease. There are many types of heart diseases, for example, congenital (genetic) heart defects, rheumatic (infectious) heart diseases, and cardio-vascular diseases (CVD). The two former types are not discussed here. The most common and preventable one is CVD.

Heart diseases are the number one cause of death among people in the US[6] and industrialized nations. Although people with heart diseases live longer than they used to, the number of heart diseases diagnosed have not declined. In fact, it has been increasing even when there are fewer smokers.

Current common risk factors are identified below by the Centers for Disease Control and Prevention (CDC). Many risk factors are related to metabolic processes in the body, but that fact is not reflected in the many treatments, which usually identify and attempt to treat the symptoms of the risk factors individually. There are medications to treat high blood pressure, medications to treat high cholesterol, and insulin to treat high glucose levels (diabetes). All these treatments address risk factors or symptoms, not the cause of heart disease. It is not making the heart or the body healthier because they are not cures. Drugs will have unwanted side effects and may impede the healing process. Addressing the whole body and the metabolic processes with food choices and lifestyle is a better approach but prescription drugs are more often used.

According to the CDC, the following are risk factors for heart disease[7]:

High blood cholesterol
Diabetes
High blood pressure
Overweight and obesity
Smoking
Unhealthy diet (Eating foods high in fat, cholesterol, and sodium)
Physical inactivity
Excessive alcohol use

It is fair to say that current care with identifying the risk factors and making common recommendations have not reduced the numbers of chronic metabolic diseases, including CVD. Either the current recommendations are not entirely correct, or people are not following the guidelines, or both. The 'Unhealthy diet' risk factor above is disappointing in terms of identifying the items to avoid. A new way to look at heart disease is that it is a result of metabolic disorder, like insulin resistance, diabetes, and obesity. They are related to each other and to the foods we eat. Note how sugar or flour consumption did not make it to the list above, when there is more than enough evidence to support it. Sugar and refined grains cause inflammation and high blood pressure. The AHA has provided sugar intake limits (see Chapter 2), which should be adhered to, but general wisdom with "moderate" sugar consumption prevails, which leaves most people thinking that the amount doesn't matter much, and that fat, salt, calories, and cholesterol are to be blamed for heart conditions.

Dietary cholesterol has been unfairly treated. Current science confirms that having a high HDL component of cholesterol is more important than having a low total cholesterol level. This is true with regards to our general health and heart health. Common wisdom blames heart disease on dietary fat and cholesterol. This idea came from the works published by Ancel Keys, A book titled *Eat Well and Stay Well*, published in 1959, and the Seven Counties Study (lead by Keys), started in 1958 and published in 1978. The book became a best seller and provided the answer to a current health problem in America. Middle-aged men were suffering heart attacks. The book popularized the "diet heart hypothesis," stating that a diet high in saturated fats will result in high cholesterol and eventually, heart disease. There was no scientific data to prove this, but it was simple enough for people to understand. The book *The Cholesterol Myths: Exposing the Fallacy that Saturated Fat and Cholesterol Cause Heart Disease,* by Uffe Ravnskov, MD/PHD (2000) is recommended reading for more information about this topic.

How Keys assumed that saturated fats, which have been in our food supply for thousands of years, could be more harmful than sugar, a processed substance, has a lot to do with the word "fat." Dietary fat was thought to go directly to our bodies, create heart disease by clogging our arteries, and also make us fat. Cholesterol, a vital substance involved in inflammation and healing, was accused of being the cause of heart and vascular disease due to its presence in the afflicted location. These assumptions are too simplistic but convincing.

The Seven Countries Study was the first multi-country epidemiological study. Epidemiology works with gathered data to look for patterns of behavior that may affect the population or one's health. Collected data are observational, not facts, and does not prove any hypothesis. The results published are not helpful for many reasons. The study may have established some correlation but not causation. The study made no distinction between trans-fat and natural saturated fats. The study conducted in twenty-two countries was reduced to seven because the other fifteen did not support the hypothesis. In the years of the study, smoking was prevalent and was not considered to be a major cause of lung cancer or heart disease. Sugar consumption in the population sampled was not considered. No randomized control trials were conducted to confirm that dietary fat and cholesterol cause heart disease, and if there were, the results were never published.

During the study period, only total cholesterol can be measured, the components of cholesterol have not been identified because the technology to measure them was not available. Major components of total lipids, high-density lipoprotein (HDL), triglycerides, or the two types of low-density lipoprotein (LDL) provide us with more information. Although LDL is thought to be the bad cholesterol, it is the small dense LDL that has negative effect on the body, not the large buoyant LDL, which is considered to be neutral.

The advice to eat less salt, less saturated fat, less cholesterol, and more whole grain is still being given out today to prevent heart disease. Heart disease is still a major cause of death. Although Keys was on to the right idea that eating well keeps us healthy, he was already convinced of his theory and led us away from identifying the real culprits. His influence, although not entirely science-based, was so powerful in the nutrition field and politics that those who challenged him suffered possible career suicide. One in particular was John Yudkin, who wrote *Pure White and Deadly,* published in 1972. Yudkin believed that refined sugar was the cause of many ailments, including heart disease. Although this hypothesis is not new in nutrition science, it was discredited and ridiculed by Keys and his colleagues.

In 1961, the American Heart Association (AHA) advised Americans to eat food that is low in saturated fat and cholesterol to protect them from heart disease. When this hypothesis was adopted and recommended to the public, it became the unfortunate catalyst that drove people to seek no or low-fat foods, indulge in sugar-rich carbohydrates, and deprive themselves of healthy fats. The food industry responded by producing more low-fat foods. To make low-fat foods palatable, more sugar or HFCS was added. Americans are now eating more refined carbs, more sugar in order to avoid fat. In addition, sugared sodas, an occasional treat, became an everyday drink in households because of availability and price.

Since high cholesterol was thought to cause heart disease, total blood cholesterol level reduction became the goal of the medical and pharmaceutical industries. Many people were placed on cholesterol reducing medication like statin to lower their cholesterol levels. Currently, science has demonstrated that reducing cholesterol is ineffective in reducing heart disease. Reducing total cholesterol or LDL amount does not always protect the heart. A high HDL level is considered protective against heart disease. Lowering cholesterol with drugs can actually can harm the body with unintended side effects.

Foods, such as seeds, nuts, eggs, fatty meats, and seafood, high in natural fats and omega-3 fatty acids with EPA and DHA should be recommended for heart health since they are known to increase the beneficial HDL cholesterol. With this information, cholesterol-lowering medications should not be prioritized in routine treatment, except in few rare cases, like familial hypercholesterolemia, which is a genetic disorder, resulting in extremely high cholesterol levels that require fat avoidance and medication.

Having high blood pressure (hypertension) is a major risk factor for heart and vascular disease. This condition put unnecessary strain on the heart and blood vessels. Many are told to limit salt and take medication to reduce blood pressure. Limiting salt will lower blood pressure by a small amount but may affect cellular signaling if electrolytes are too low. Lowering sugar and flour intake is more beneficial by reducing uric acid, which has been identified as a major cause of hypertension—a major driver of heart disease and stroke. Dietary and lifestyle changes can be effective in reducing hypertension by optimizing the whole body. Taking blood pressure medication aimed at reducing blood pressure does not cure the cause of high blood pressure. It temporarily reduces it, give you unwanted side effects and leave you dependent on medication that is managing your symptoms.

Another important factor that impact our heart and vascular health is the hormone insulin. When our diets are full of sugar and refined flour, we produce insulin to manage the elevated glucose that unfortunately follows. When insulin is chronically elevated as with insulin resistance or type 2 diabetes conditions, it induces growth which may include the lining of the blood vessels, or endothelial cells contributing to high blood pressure since the diameter of the blood vessels are reduced. Treating the cause of insulin resistance or excess insulin to optimize the heart and blood vessels should be considered, not just maintaining proper glucose levels with insulin.

Stress reduction or management is important for heart and overall health. Prolonged stress increases cortisol, an important hormone that is associated with the "fight or flight" mode of the nervous system. High cortisol levels can create chronic inflammation that may lead to high blood pressure, which is not good for the blood vessels or the heart. Addressing the source of stress and learning to manage it will help lower the cortisol levels and reduce inflammation.

Cardio-vascular disease (CVD) is associated with the quality of our blood, blood vessels, heart, and brain, which are intricately linked. Food choices and lifestyle have major impact on your heart and health. This message is not being adequately recommended. Taking medication to address the risk factors may not be the correct treatment but this is usually the first thought of "preventative" medicine. Usually, drugs are prescribed to treat risk factors of heart disease and also to treat side effects.

All medications have unintended consequences and our bodies are not designed to rely on them for health in the long term. We have been led to believe that we need science and medication to heal us. This may be true in cases of trauma, birth defects, or infections, but for people not suffering from severe conditions, we can heal ourselves.

We need to see our health as a body of cooperating cells and organs. Optimizing the metabolic function with diet and lifestyle choices will heal the heart and the whole body. Medications, if needed, should be considered for short-term use with proper benefits to risk analysis.

10. Toxins

We are exposed to toxins through the air we breathe, the foods we eat, through our skin, and from normal cellular metabolism. Anything dangerous to our bodies is eliminated through various means, with the help of the respiratory, lymphatic, digestive, or circulatory system. The body determines the threat level and prioritizes removal of harmful invaders over normal routine functions.

When toxins accumulate and are not disposed of properly, they will affect our physical or mental health. Many conditions can cause this, either frequent exposures to toxins or impaired ability to detoxify. One of the major causes of inadequate toxin removal is unhealthy liver. Other causes include impaired kidneys, lack of glucose control, or leaky gut, which will induce inflammation.

The liver has many important functions, an important one is to trap harmful materials and help the body remove them. This will not happen efficiently when the liver is clogged with fat deposited as a result of too much sugar or fructose in the diet. Toxins, when produced by the body (as a by-product of energy metabolism) and from the environment, air, food, and drugs, need to be removed to keep us safe and functional.

To optimize health, we can lower our exposure to any known toxic chemicals, heavy metals, pesticides, and herbicides (glyphosate) by avoiding them. Many chemicals are known carcinogens, causing cancer when exposed to them either frequently or in high doses. Some chemicals are carcinogenic but have not been thoroughly investigated so have not made it to the "dangerous for humans" list. Many farm workers have poor health and cancer due to the regular handling of pesticides and herbicides.

Some chemicals to avoid: chlorine bleach, triclosin, paraben, sodium laureth sulfate (SLS), oxybenzene. Phthalates, a family of industrial chemicals, used to soften polyvinyl chloride (PVC) plastic and as solvents in cosmetics and other consumer products, can damage the liver, kidneys, lungs, and reproductive system. Exposure to these chemicals is usually through the skin, in the form of detergents, soaps, shampoos, lotions, make-up, or sunscreens. Not only are these chemicals bad for our bodies, they are not good for the environment. Many soaps, shampoos, and laundry and dishwashing detergents are now made without these harmful chemicals.

The Environmental Working Group (EWG.org) provides information and data to help the public identify and avoid certain chemicals that are known to be harmful. They also publish a list of vegetables and fruits that are commonly exposed to pesticides and herbicides, and should be eaten organic when possible.

Some harmful chemicals are called endocrine disruptors, which mimic hormones and disrupt the functioning of the endocrine system, the communications system in the body, by incorrectly binding with estrogen receptors. For example, BPA (bisphenol A) was recently used in plastic, like baby bottles, water bottles, and many household items, but has since been banned due to harmful effects. Avoid the use of plastic to limit exposure to questionable chemicals. Glass and metal are better options for food and drink containers.

BHA (butylated hydroxyanisole) and BHT (butylated hydroxytoluene) are closely related synthetic antioxidants used as preservatives. According to the EWG, multiple studies have linked BHT to tumor growth, hormone disruption, and reproductive harm. BHA, a preservative that's chemically similar, is a known carcinogen according to California state scientists. Both these chemicals have been subjected to severe restrictions in the European Union (EU), Canada, and Japan. Even so, many popular foods in the US contain either BHT or BHA. According to EWG's Food Scores database, 2,830 products contain BHT, including popular cereals like Cinnamon Toast Crunch and Froot Loops.

Historically dentists would advise people to avoid too much sugar to prevent cavities. With the use of fluoride in toothpaste and water supply, cavities became less common but not eradicated. Fluoride is a toxin, a byproduct chemical of aluminum processing. In very small amounts, it can help slow the cavity formation process on teeth. It is the amount put into our water supply that is being questioned by many. Too much ingested is toxic, especially for growing children.

Being aware of toxins to avoid and reading labels is important since government regulations are slow. For example, we were exposed to lead paint, lead pipes, asbestos, and second-hand cigarette smoke for many decades before it was determined to be harmful. Glyphosate is banned in Europe but is still widely sold and used in the US, especially in commercial agriculture. The US is behind the European nations in banning harmful chemicals to protect the population due to the lack of resources and power in the regulating agencies like the Environmental Protecting Agency (EPA) and U.S. Food and Drug Administration (FDA). Strong corporate influence and "revolving door" practices in these agencies and corporations have prioritized corporate profit over safety of people.

Don't let the marketing industry sell you harmful substances that may hurt you or the earth. Less harsh chemical is better when it comes to cleaning dishes, laundry, homes, and our bodies. We have to protect our microbiome that is protecting us. Use environmentally safe cleaning products along with sunscreens, moisturizers, soaps, and shampoos without known toxins. With more chemical exposures, our bodies will need to work harder. This condition can weaken our immune system.

In addition to avoiding toxins, we can help our bodies detoxify by eating whole foods with fiber, healthy fats, and plenty of water. Getting adequate sleep will help detox the brain. Sweating is a good way to get rid of harmful substances through our skin. This can be induced by frequent and rigorous exercise or even frequent use of saunas or steam rooms.

11. Supplements

When we are eating a variety of nutritious foods, sleeping well, actively moving, and getting adequate exposure to sunlight, we should have all we need to thrive. In reality, our diets are not ideal, we are exposed to toxins daily, and we don't get enough sunlight exposure to make enough vitamin D.

Vitamin D is a vital steroid hormone and not a vitamin by definition. It was misnamed due to our lack of knowledge when it was discovered, but it will always be referred to as a "vitamin." It is a very important and needed throughout the body and serves many vital functions, including the immune system, bone formation, heart and brain health. Without sufficient amounts, we can suffer symptoms like depression, allergies, skin conditions, weak bones and muscles, arthritis, hypertension, or inflammation. The energy (UVB) from the sun is absorbed through our skin, produces chemicals that are transported and converted to vitamin D. It is called a fat-soluble vitamin since it needs fat (cholesterol) for processing and transporting. It is stored in the body, unlike water-soluble vitamins that is excreted from the body daily. Overdosing or too much vitamin D is unlikely but deficiency is very common.

The lack of sun exposure and use of sunscreen are preventing us from getting an optimal amount of vitamin D, unlike our ancestors who spent most of their time outdoors. Supplementation with vitamin D3(cholecalciferol) is highly recommended unless you live near the equator and spend a lot of time outdoors. Blood lab work can confirm your level to see if and how much supplementation is needed. Taking 1000 IU to 5000 IU daily is common even for those in the low normal range.

Omega-3 fatty acids (with EPA and DHA) are important for heart and brain health. It is not prevalent in the current western diet. In nature, omega-3 fatty acids can be obtained from flax/chia/hemp seeds, fish, caviar, and grass-fed beef. Most agree that supplementation is recommended to maintain health. These fatty acids are associated with healing, repair and have anti-inflammation properties.

Minerals are important and are found in whole foods. Some common minerals are magnesium, potassium, calcium, and sodium. There are some that we need in small trace amounts, like zinc, manganese, and copper. They are vital for optimal health. It should be noted that if our diet is high in sugar and refined grains, we can deplete our bodies of minerals especially magnesium because minerals are needed to buffer the effect of acid producing grains and sugar. Our bodies need to maintain an optimal PH level and will pull minerals out of our bones if it does not have enough. To increase magnesium naturally, we can eat plenty of nuts like almonds or cashews and plenty of green leafy vegetables.

Probiotics are common supplements that may be considered to optimize gut health. It is years of eating diverse and nutritious whole foods with plenty of soluble and insoluble fibers that lead to a balanced gut microbiome, which aids in many functions including digestion, brain health, metabolic health, and immunity. Many times, our guts become imbalanced due to poor diet, lack of sleep, stress, hormone insufficiency, or taking too many rounds of antibiotics. For these and other conditions, we may require a stronger "resetting" of the gut. There have been many strains of bacteria that have been identified as healthy for our guts and will survive our stomach acid when ingested. There are many strains that have been identified with poor health. The goal is not to eradicate all the "bad" microbes, but to keep them in check with many other helpful strains.

This field is active and we may in the future treat viral infections with bacteria or eliminate bacterial infections with another strain of bacteria instead of killing them all with antibiotics (which originally was derived from mold microbes).

Obtaining enough nutrients from a variety of foods can help prevent deficiencies. Scurvy and rickets are results of severe depletion of vitamins C and D. Although these conditions are not common now, there are other health conditions related to deficiencies. For example, a lack of vitamin B12 is associated with many symptoms like fatigue and even mental disorder symptoms. A lack of iodine can lead to hypothyroidism. Nutritional deficiency is often overlooked, and should be part of identifying possible causes of illness.

Taking a quality multiple vitamins and minerals daily is a good way to insure that you are not deficient.

12. Type 2 Diabetes

Before the 1980s, type 2 diabetes was not that common. It was called adult onset diabetes or type 2 to distinguish it from type 1, which is found mostly in children and is incurable. Type 2 diabetes was rare for adults and even rarer for children. Today, it is very common for middle age and older adults and more prevalent in children. No one is surprised when they are told they or someone they know have the disease. There are many drugs, devices, magazines, products, and supplements available and marketed to diabetics. We seem to have developed a resistance to the fact that we are living in an epidemic of non-infectious disease.

Since the diabetes epidemic coincided with the obesity epidemic, it was mostly assumed that type 2 diabetes was the result of being overweight or obese. It was believed that being overweight leads to type 2 diabetes. This assumption provided the simple answer to the problem and also the solution. Healthcare professionals and the general public agree that people are eating too many calories and not exercising enough. The solution is simple. They just need to lose weight.

Fear of gaining weight and being fat lead many to eat low or no fat foods. Sugar has fewer calories than fat, so was considered to be acceptable in moderation. In addition the "heart health hypothesis" has driven fear of heart disease into people. Avoiding fat and cholesterol to keep our hearts healthy means eating less fat, less whole animals, fewer calories, and more carbohydrates like whole grains and sugar.

This common wisdom of "simple" solution failed. The assumption that we can control our weight with calories or exercise is wrong. The assumption that natural saturated fat and cholesterol causes heart disease is wrong. Blaming the population and not the health advice or treatment is convenient. It is interesting to note that this problem is worldwide and not just for the overweight. Although more overweight people have this condition, many thin people also suffer metabolic diseases. In Asian countries, type 2 diabetes is prevalent in the last several decades where obesity is not.

Type 2 diabetes occurs when the body cannot regulate the glucose level in the blood. A high fasting glucose level is usually how one is diagnosed. Obesity is not the cause of diabetes or vice versa. They are both metabolic disorders, not just due to the consumption of high-calorie foods and sedentary life. The metabolic disorder occurs when the hormone insulin is ineffective, constantly high, or both high and ineffective.

When we eat foods high in carbohydrates especially refined flour, our glucose level will spike, which will require insulin to be released to remove excess glucose from the blood and into cells where they can be used for energy. Typically, our bodies will do what it can to normalize us. By storing excess glucose and fructose as fat, it has temporarily saved us from high blood sugar, but in time, we will run out of places to store this energy if the glucose input is too large or too frequent. Our bodies reluctantly store it where it should not be, in our organs. The liver, kidneys, or pancreas may become damaged with excess fat and will not function properly. With suboptimal organs, our body cannot control blood glucose levels, heal, convert food to energy, or eliminate toxins efficiently.

The pancreas secretes the hormone insulin to manage the elevated glucose level. When elevated glucose is detected frequently, the insulin level in the body is also elevated. A condition called hyper-insulinemia is present when insulin levels are always high. Cells will protect themselves, from constant exposure to insulin by down-regulating the insulin receptors. When the cells become immune to insulin, a condition known as insulin resistance, has taken place, and the body now needs more insulin to deliver energy and regulate the blood. The insensitivity of insulin drives higher insulin production and levels. This cycle becomes problematic if not stopped.

An important factor in glucose management is the fact that insulin can't force glucose into cells that are already full of glucose so it remains in the blood stream. Until there is room, insulin cannot do its job but will keep on trying because it is very important to regulate blood glucose. We either have to slow or stop the flow of glucose coming into the body or use up what we have, or both to help this process.

High-sustained levels of insulin are not good for the body since it is a fat storage hormone, meant for intermittent use. There are many problems associated with constant high insulin levels. Our kidneys will not excrete excess sodium, which may result in hypertension. Our body will not use fat for fuel. To unlock the door to fat stores, insulin level has to be normal. Insulin is a hormone, a chemical messenger that interacts with other hormones. When it dominates the body, it reduces the effectiveness of other hormones. By design, it will hoard energy and will not let the body use stored fat.

Diabetes is our body's way of telling us that it needs help. With too much sugar in the blood left unchecked, the high glucose and high insulin levels will impair organs that are being nourished by this sugary blood. This can lead to blindness, kidney failure, nerve damage, or amputation of limbs. This is why medication like metformin or insulin is prescribed, to keep blood glucose levels in check. What is ironic is that using insulin to treat high glucose level also causes weight gain. Patients are told to lose weight, while given hormones that drive up weight gain that makes diabetes worse, so they need more insulin. This is how the disease becomes progressively worse.

The current diabetes treatment of using drugs or insulin to normalize the glucose is not fixing the problem. It is fixing one of the many symptoms of metabolic disorder. Figuring out how to correct the source of the metabolic disorder should be discussed. Most people are unaware of what this condition is, why they have it, and how to reverse or prevent it. They often blame genetics or bad luck and think they can't do anything about it.

Before the discovery of insulin in the 1920s, treatment for type 2 diabetes included diet restrictions. Patients were discouraged from eating foods that drive up glucose levels, like starches, bread, pasta, and sugar. After insulin was successfully used on type 1 diabetic patients, doctors started using insulin on type 2 diabetic patients. They thought that with insulin, patients could generally eat whatever they want and manage the glucose level with drugs. They may not be aware of the harmful effects of too much insulin on the body.

We deserve to have correct information and choices. Unfortunately, the healthcare industry considers type 2 diabetes to be a progressive disease, and does not strongly promote treatment options that can cure the patient. They are not telling the patients to abstain from sugar and foods that drive glucose levels up. Patients are allowed to continue to eat whole grains, less fat, count carbs, and take medication or insulin to "manage" their glucose levels. This treatment will invoke the progressiveness of this condition because the food advice is wrong. There is less chance of cure down this road. Most people don't know that this is a choice. There are other options. In many cases, type 2 diabetes can be reversed or managed without medication. It involves eating whole foods and not eating processed foods (sugar and flour). It may involve regular exercise and fasting to get the body sensitive to insulin again. It is not easy to do, but it will improve the quality of life and increase longevity.

The Diabetes Code by Dr. Jason Fung explains the disease and the ways to reverse it. He is one of many doctors who wondered why conventional treatments were not making people better but worse. He found a better way to heal and empower his patients. You may not have heard about it because there is no money to be made when the treatment does not include any medication. No pharmaceutical company is going to help spread this information. Sadly, there are currently doctors who are promoting bariatric surgery, which carries significant risks for patients who are obese and diabetic. This type of treatment is expensive, damaging to the body, and not always effective. Have they tried the inexpensive natural treatments? Fasting would be a less traumatic and cost nothing. Many people have reversed their pre-diabetes and type 2 diabetes with dietary changes and intermittent fasting. They are not limiting calories or fat, but limiting carbs, and refined flour. They don't go hungry because they can eat most whole foods with satiating fats. This information and advice need to be in mainstream healthcare.

Another condition, previously thought to be rare, is a form of pre-diabetes. It is called reactive hypoglycemia. It is when a high spike in glucose levels is followed by a crash to abnormally low glucose levels. For these individuals, the symptoms of low blood sugar are not pleasant (headache, fatigue, inability to think clearly) and will drive them to find food to elevate the glucose level, and this cycle continues. It is theorized that individuals with this condition will become diabetic if not diagnosed and presented with a better lifestyle and food choice. A book called *A Sugar Nation* by Jeff O'Connell explores his pre-diabetic condition that he faced along with loosing his father to type 2 diabetes. Detailing his journey into the world of type 2 diabetes, Jeff found little help from mainstream healthcare or even the American Diabetes Association (ADA), who were supposed to be experts in the field. The industry has already assumed that he will get worse and need drug therapy. With his own research, he discovered a diet and lifestyle change that stabilized his glucose level and reversed his condition.

There are many who have taken the path less travelled and can attest to its outcome. They took control of their health and saved themselves. How do we connect those people to the ones recently diagnosed? It would be better for us to prevent them and ourselves from being diagnosed in the first place. It is hard to change the norm, especially when money is being made in many industries involved with treatment. We need to advocate prevention and cure. It is necessary for longevity and health span improvement.

Recently, there are new electronic devices on the market that will monitor your blood glucose level continuously (CGM) by incorporating a patch that is attached to your arm. The patch detects the glucose level and relays the information to your phone or meter. This is helpful in providing continuous data in almost real-time on how your blood is affected by food, medication, and activities. Currently it is being used to help with insulin or drug management for diagnosed diabetic patients. The cost for this type of device is high and insurance coverage may not be available or be limited. In the future, this may change and we can all benefit from using it as a preventative tool.

13. Calories

A Calorie (kcal) is the amount of energy needed to raise the temperature of 1 kilogram of water 1 degree Celsius.

Basically, a calorie is how much heat energy is given off when burning a sample of a substance, like protein, fat, alcohol, or carbohydrate in a calorimeter.

It was determined and generally accepted that burning the following items produces:

Carbohydrate	=	4Kcal/gram
Protein	=	4Kcal/gram
Fat	=	9Kcal/gram
Alcohol	=	7Kcal/gram

Typically, the Atwater system equation is used to determine total calorie in food based on the above data.

The formula:

Energy (in Kcal) = 4 × (protein mass in grams + carbohydrate mass in grams) + 9 × mass of fat in grams.

The above equation is commonly used to calculate calorie contents of food products. This is a man-made concept to quantify food and energy. It may have some merits in certain scientific application, but it is not always helpful when it comes to defining human health and nutrition.

We have all heard the word calorie and assume we know what a calorie is. It is the energy in food that is transferred to us when we eat. When we move and exercise, we use up the energy. So, we gain weight if we take in more calories than we expend. And losing weight would be the opposite. This idea of calorie balance is misleading. It assumes that we can control how we spend our calories or energy. Moving our bodies or exercising may require us to use energy but this is a small amount of energy compared to the energy we spend each day just being alive. Our automatically regulated systems are complex and do not have a simple linear relationship with our caloric input. There is no conservation of energy rule that applies to the biochemistry of the human body.

The concept of calories in nutrition science is dated. It was adopted as if it were a scientific discovery. It is not. It was an attempt to understand and measure food energy, and relate it to human health and nutrition. Controlling calorie input and output to change body weight may sometimes work, but not because of the calorie equation. Our bodies are far more complex; we have redundant systems, and are adaptive to optimizing our resources. Growth, height, muscle mass, fat formation, and fat storage are not controlled by calories. They are regulated by many things, including genetics, nutrient sensors, and many various communicating hormones.

The calorie energy equation assumes that energy is stored in the human body the same way no matter where it is from. Unlike the calorimeter, our bodies do not combust or burn food to just generate heat. It is also not a closed system. Food is digested by mechanical and biochemical means. Energy and nutrients are extracted and processed in a highly complex system to maintain many vital functions, body heat, heart rate, blood pressure, brain activity, and muscle movements. We have redundant or back up fuel sources (glycogen and fat) to maintain this intricate system. To say that we can control our weight by adjusting calorie input is too simplistic. All calories are not the same in the human body. A calorie tells you very little about the composition of the food, how or what we will do with the food. It tells us that if we put that food in a calorimeter and burn it by igniting it, we will get heat, energy, or "calorie." How this concept is associated with health and used in the field of nutrition shows how little progress is made in this field. Many thoughtful scientists and writers have fallen into this "calorie" trap and use it interchangeably with energy. This vague concept has been impeding our understanding of the role our diet plays in health.

Food has a complex composition and is commonly reduced to glucose, amino acids, fatty acids, or fiber. All these components are being used differently by our bodies and also by the microorganisms in our intestines. Feeding our bodies and our microbes with needed substances help us maintain health and has little to do with calories. What a calorie can tell you is the amount of food you have. For example, two apples will have more calories than one apple, but saying 100 calories of an apple is equal to 100 calories of a donut is misleading. It may be a true statement, but it does not equate to how our body uses energy or nutrients from each. A calorie is not relevant or understood by our bodies. We don't have calorie sensors. We have nutrient sensors located at various points in our digestive system. These sensors help us with digestion and communications with our various energy and metabolic needs.

Food provides energy and nutrients. Calorie is how much heat a substance produces when burned. The two things can overlap but do not equate to each other. Wood and alcohol can be burned to generate heat but that does not make them food. We need to let go of this misleading concept that calories are important for health. This idea is so pervasive and ingrained in our thinking. The food industries have successfully used it to justify and promote their products.

Does the weight of food relate to how good it is for us? A calorie is a measurement, just like the measuring of how much food weighs or what temperature food is. It can only give us one aspect of a substance.

It took many years to change the minds of astrologers and scientists before they can accept that the sun does not revolve around the earth. Accepting that "calorie" is misleading and not meaningful when applied to nutrition and health will also take time.

14. Pharmaceuticals

Pharmaceutical companies have had many great successes. With vaccines, antibiotics, insulin, pain management drugs, etc., lives have been saved and extended. Unfortunately, they also had numerous failures. Many drugs have been approved and then taken off the market by due to severe adverse reactions and deaths. Drug makers provide doctors with treatment options for many ailments and diseases. They provide tools for healthcare in aiding our repair and recovery. The positive contribution of drug companies to healthcare has been tremendous.

In order to compete and survive in a competitive market, drug makers need to continually develop new drugs or improve current drugs. That is where the money is, in new drug patents and sales. Recently, advertising products to the general population has been an effective marketing strategy. Selling more products is the goal, not always curing diseases or helping us stay healthy. The problem with an industry that makes multi-billion dollars is that they have the resources to influence government, research, healthcare, and medical programs to promote their products.

Symptom management is big money. For example, there are many products aimed at managing headaches, migraines, or the common cold. Unfortunately a cure for the cold is not quite there yet. Management and cure are very different. We need to realize that what we are prescribed may not be curing us. All pharmaceutical drugs have side effects and can hurt us, especially with long-term use. It may impede our body's healing process. This is also true of risk factor modification drugs. For example, when cholesterol level was thought (and still believed) to be a major risk factor for heart disease, many people were placed on cholesterol-lowering medication, like Statin. This is an example of taking medication to treat a risk factor for a disease, not the disease it self. Risk factors are not the cause of, but may contribute to the disease. New information has negated this risk factor and the advice to lower cholesterol has not changed much. As it turned out, for most people, this preemptive medication did not reduce heart disease but gave people muscle pain, headache, digestive issues, and fatigue. From total cholesterol lowering to LDL lowering, drugs have been the focus of mitigating this risk factor. There are two types of LDL, one being large and buoyant, the other small and dense. The drugs do not reduce the small dense, more harmful LDL. The overall cholesterol may go down, but does not correlate with healthier blood or heart.

We sometimes forget how precious and resilient our bodies are. We do not need to become reliant on medications to solve all our illnesses and discomforts because we can heal. Pain is a diagnostic tool. From it, we know something is wrong. We can find the cause and fix the problem. Painkillers do not make the source of the pain go away but can help us get through trauma recovery. When we have a fever, our body generates more body heat as part of the immune response to get rid of unwanted invading foreigners. Having a fever makes us tired, to sleep and rest while we heal. To many, fever is a sickness but it is actually a tool we have to heal. It is a symptom of our body dealing with an infection. With fever reducer medication, we bring our temperature down and feel better, and we don't rest, as we should. This process is not working with the body but against it. Our ability to efficiently fight the infection is reduced when we take away its natural defense. There are times where an infection is getting out of control and we may need to reduce body temperature or take antibiotics, but too often we reach for the drugs right away because we want to heal instantly. Letting our bodies heal naturally is good practice for our immune system. Not taking more medication than necessary is the right step toward keeping our bodies optimal. All medication, even aspirin, have unintended consequences on our fragile biological ecosystem. Overuse of common pain relievers, acetaminophens and ibuprofens has been blamed for poor liver and gut health.

Currently, medications aimed at treating mental health disorders like depression, attention deficit and hyperactivity disorder (ADHD), and anxiety, are commonly prescribed. Due to the marketing of the drugs and social acceptance, more people are being diagnosed and getting help. Sadly, most of the help are medication-based. These conditions are symptoms, which are treated as though they were diseases. There may be valid reasons to try medication when all else has failed, but more people are placed on medication aimed at eliminating the symptoms or to fix chemical imbalances in the brain.

People are led to believe that they are chemically imbalanced or "off" and need to be corrected to feel normal, according to Kelly Brogan MD, a board-certified psychiatrist, who studied cognitive neuroscience at MIT and received an MD from Weill Cornell Medical College. She wrote *A Mind of Your Own* and *Own Your Self*. Doctors, like herself, were taught to prescribe antidepressants but were never taught to wean anyone off. She experienced this difficulty when many patients came to her, trying to get off the medications when they were trying to start a family. Her research on antidepressants and brain health lead her to the conclusion that little benefits are obtained but the side effects and addictions are much worse. It is appalling how much is prescribed without proper risk to benefit analysis. Any physician with no experience in mental disorders or neuroscience background can prescribe these drugs. These psychotropic drugs are designed to alleviate symptoms.

These symptoms should alert us to what is not going right in our daily lives, whether it's our diet, stress, perceived stress, or current or past trauma. We need to listen and look for clues to find the true causes and heal. People on these medications are not cured of any affliction but may become addicts and suffer physically and mentally when trying to get off the drugs. They were not told these drugs were addictive. Many have been on it for decades.

The use of Selective Serotonin Reuptake Inhibitors (SSRI) drugs like Zoloft was thought to help keep the neurotransmitter serotonin level from diminishing by blocking its reuptake to combat psychiatric disorders like depression or anxiety. This chemical imbalance theory no longer describes the problem that the drugs were supposed to fix. Serotonin is not the only neurotransmitter and having more does not fix the problem and will affect other aspects of cell communication. Serotonin is not the problem or the fix, as the drug companies want you to think. The chemical and electrical signaling of neurons and gut communication are more complex, but healing is possible. Many neurological disorders like depression, ADHD, and anxiety have been linked to brain inflammation, which can often be cured by treating the whole body. When these symptoms are present, the brain is responding to some internal or external forces that are driving inflammation. Changing the chemistry with drugs does not usually heal or improve functions, but has unintended consequences. Some early positive effects of these antidepressant drugs have been attributed to the placebo effect or mild reduction of inflammation. Dr. Brogan does not believe in the effectiveness of antidepressant drug therapy. Her research brought much insight into the healing of the human body and mind. In her current practice, she no longer prescribes any antidepressant drugs. She feels that our bodies are better off going through the natural process, which may involve pain due to various causes like personal loss or trauma, than avoiding it with mind-numbing drugs. It may be difficult, but we can heal naturally using our own tools.

Antidepressants or mood disorder drugs are symptom management drugs, not intended to cure us of any disease and make it harder for us to heal. The same is true for drugs like Ritalin or Adderall in the treatment of ADHD for both adults and children. In some cases, short-term use may help, but long-term goal of drug free treatment should be considered to truly heal.

Emerging science has established strong connections between gut health, metabolic health, and brain health. The book *Brain Maker* by Dr. Perlmutter has good information relating to this rapidly expanding field. Many things influence the health of our gut, including food, drugs, exposure to toxins, and even lack of exposure to beneficial microbes. In turn, gut health affects both our cells' metabolic health and cell communication and functionality in the brain. It is common to find people suffering mental health issues such as depression or anxiety, also suffer gastrointestinal issues. This is a multidirectional process that will affect the whole body. When threatened negatively, the body will respond with inflammation in an attempt to heal.

The discovery of antibiotics has saved numerous lives from bacterial infections. Before this discovery, we did not know about our gut microbiome or how important its collective functions are within our bodies. The current misuse of antibiotics on humans, as well as the overuse on farm animals, has created strains of drug-resistant bacteria. These super bugs may become a much larger problem if we don't address these issues. There is already a problem with the pathogenic strain clostridium difficile (C. diff). Many have died from this infection, which is resistant to antibiotics. This is a massive problem in hospitals and nursing homes. Our bodies are affected by the killing of harmful bugs as the helpful bugs are destroyed as well. When people are subjected to multiple rounds of antibiotics, the health of their gut microbiome is decimated. The overall health of the gut, which is our major source of immunity are diminished. Doctors need to be more selective when deciding if we really need to be on antibiotics. Many question the frequent routine use of prophylactic antibiotics. In addition, we should remember that they do not work on viral or fungal infections. Unfortunately, even if we don't use antibiotics, we may be exposed to them through our food and water supplies.

Insulin, a necessary human hormone, was discovered and later produced in the 1920s to successfully treat type 1 diabetes, a condition where the body (pancreas) cannot produce insulin and will eventually die because food cannot be converted to energy. Type 1 diabetes is rare and not curable, but with insulin and good glucose control, people can live a full life. This was the life saving miracle of the synthesized insulin when used properly. Too much insulin can induce coma and death. Many years later, insulin became an option for treating type 2 diabetes as well. An assumption was made that these two conditions were alike (high glucose level), so treatments are similar. Injected insulin is used to control the glucose level in the blood. In reality, type 2 diabetes is very different from type 1. Insulin production in the body of type 2 diabetics is not impaired. In fact, it is too high or ineffective. Using more insulin to decrease glucose levels in the blood is a temporary fix, which adds to the unhealthy insulin level in the body. The obvious question should be, why are the cells not receptive to insulin? Are they already full of glucose to take any more in or are they down regulating their receptors to protect themselves from over exposure to insulin? Again, this treatment is taking care of the high glucose level, which is important, but the source of the problem still exists and a cure is not happening if the symptoms are just managed.

We need to be aware of why we are prescribed drugs, for how long, and if there are other treatment options. For all of us, having a drug-free life is preferred.

15. Inflammation and Infection

Inflammation is a biological process in which our bodies are in repair mode. When subjected to trauma, our immune system and healing process are activated. This process is part of the miracle you see when you cut or scrape yourself, and when your skin becomes swollen, scabs, and eventually heals. This acute inflammation is necessary for healing. It is the chronic, or inflammation that does not end but lingers, that can harm us. Our bodies cannot be in this repair mode continuously. Inflammation can affect the brain, heart, lungs, intestines, nervous system, gums, or any organ. Some typical causes are smoking, drugs, allergies, toxins, sugar, stress, hormonal imbalances, low stomach acid, leaky gut, and infections. The causes are many and some are related to our metabolism. Healing starts with removing the causes. Our current health epidemic can be attributed to excessive chronic inflammation, brought on by poor diet, lifestyle, and exposures to infections or toxins. Our body's inflammatory response is another way it is trying to protect us from harm. Even if this harm may be self-caused.

Inflammation can negatively affect our ability to overcome infections. Infections can come from foreign organisms or our own bodies when organisms living on or in us become too abundant. Because this threat is a constant part of living, we have a sophisticated immune system that efficiently identifies our friends and foes. On a healthy human, our defenses are strong and most "bugs" are kept in check. When our defenses are down due to suboptimal health, we lack both the means to identify and to eradicate harmful materials. This can result in inflammation that is chronic because the body lacks the tools or the strength needed to eradicate or neutralize the infection. Sometimes, it is the opposite, our bodies are trying to eradicate harmful invaders, and instead overreact and hurt our own bodies.

Our oral health is important and a good indication of overall health. Many things, including our diet and hygiene, affect the health of our teeth and gums. Keeping our mouths healthy should be prioritized since any oral infection is a potential toxin in the blood that can lead to damages in the joints, organs, or the brain. Infection in the mouth has been linked to cognitive impairment symptoms. Treating the infection can remove some dementia-like symptoms as discussed in the book *The End to Alzheimer's Program* by Dr. Bredesen.

Many foods and certain spices are known to have anti-inflammatory properties, such as tea, turmeric, tart cherries, and omega-3 fatty acids. Sleeping and exercising are natural ways our bodies reduce inflammation and heal. Anti-inflammatory substances may help, but focusing on removing the harmful sources of chronic inflammation will be more effective in the healing process.

Conclusion

All humans living in industrialized nations are currently at risk for developing some form of chronic metabolic disease. The cluster of diseases, commonly known as metabolic syndrome, includes obesity, type 2 diabetes, insulin resistance, hypertension, cardio vascular disease, dementia, and fatty liver. They are related to each other and are affected by our food choices. Chronic metabolic diseases have been on the rise worldwide. Food affects the health and metabolism of our cells, and ultimately our whole body. The shift in our food environment, belief in the misguided calorie balance equation, and incorrect nutrition advice has left us in this dire situation.

We can stop this epidemic and promote health through knowledge and understanding. When we recognize the harmful effects of excess sugar and flour, we can make better food choices either gradually or drastically as we see fit. We are in the driver's seat when it comes to our health. What we do matter. For too long, we believed that it was genetics, luck, and that all food was good for us in a certain amount. There is no moderation when the substance is addictive and harmful to our bodies. There should be stronger recommendations and restrictions when it comes to the consumption of sugar and processed foods. Sadly, due to the profit driven nature of the food and drink industry, this is not happening. We were led to believe that fat, salt, sedentary life, and too many calories are the problems.

A rapidly expanding field of science that explores the role of our gut microbiome, has established that different microbes, their variety, and population affect our health. Optimizing our food and lifestyle will positively affect these microscopic friends and help strengthen our body and overall health.

We have to correct the misguided concept of calories. All calories are not equal, and counting them is useless. It isn't working now and hasn't worked in the past. Eating low-calorie, low-fat foods has not helped the population. Let us pull the "calorie" curtains down and see food for what it is—whole, natural, or processed. Our bodies are complex, but our health is simple. Is it so simple that we missed the obvious? Eating real whole foods, including much needed natural fats will provide us with energy, fiber, and nutrients our cells and gut microbes need to thrive. Taking sugar, refined grains, and processed foods out of our diet can solve many problems because our cells struggle with too much energy and not enough nutrients. Processed foods have crowded out whole real foods.

With lower income families, eating organic is not a priority, and when fast food is cheaper and quicker than making meals, it is not a fair choice. The government should stop subsidizing wheat, corn, and soybeans (flour, HFCS, vegetable oil) and subsidize organic farms growing pastured raised eggs/animals, vegetables and fruit. We are paying with our tax dollars through subsidies and then again at the stores by buying processed grains and junk food. The sad truth is that many are unaware of this food environment that is adversely affecting their health and the health of their children. Processed and "junk" foods are everywhere. They are made with cheap ingredients and are not good for us. Education has to be part of the solution. How do we remove the conflict of interest between government and big agriculture and food companies? How do we put people first not corporate profits? There are no easy answers, but change is needed to improve the health of the population.

Health professionals are our best option for giving advice. Except that traditionally, they have had very little training in nutrition science or functional medicine. Most of the training is to save lives, perform procedures, and prescribe pharmaceuticals. Food is not usually discussed as part of health care. We need proper nutrition and lifestyle-based preventative care that is current and aimed at keeping us healthy. Sadly, healthcare of this type is still rare due to how medical care and insurance companies are managed and regulated.

The pharmaceutical companies have the resources to advertise drugs to doctors and the general public. John Abramson stated in an article in Time magazine, "The drug companies control the 'knowledge' that informs doctors' clinical decisions. This leads to soaring pharmaceutical profits and crippling healthcare costs, while doctors have no way of knowing which therapies are more effective—or more efficient."[8] Dr. Abramson is the author of the book, *Sickening: How Big Pharma Broke American Health Care and How We Can Repair It*, and serves on the clinical faculty of Harvard Medical School, where he teaches public health policy. It is not easy for doctors to keep up with new medications and its efficiency. They rarely hear about treatment options that are free. In contrast, they are bombarded with information about new pharmaceuticals because that is where money is made.

"The US Centers for Disease Control and Prevention (CDC) estimated that by 2050, one in three US adults will have diabetes. One in eight people aged sixty-five and over currently has Alzheimer's, and that number is expected to rise to one in four within the next twenty years."[9] These numbers are scary for us and for future generations. They will inherit a diminished quality of life along with an unimaginable economic burden.

Help is needed by local and federal government agencies to make changes to our food system and environment, and in schools to educate students and families. Many in public health are working to do this, but the process is slow and may not happen due to the food industry's powerful influence.. They control the farming, processing, distribution, transportation, and the majority of shelf space in stores. This "monopoly" has served them well and any change to the status quo is an up hill battle.

Industrial farming practices erode our topsoil and contaminate the environment. We have no easy way to say no to these practices when politics and money are involved. We pay with our tax dollars, our land, and our health. There is no help coming soon from the top. We have to work our way from the bottom, starting with our purchasing power. Collectively, we can make a difference.

The good news:

The human body is a miracle. It is a part of nature and wants to thrive. The key is finding the right information, nutrition, and lifestyle to properly care for it. We have more control than we think regarding our health and longevity. Our genetics play a smaller role in chronic metabolic diseases. It is epigenetics, the interaction between our DNA and our environment. Our diet and lifestyle help to decide what genes are expressed or suppressed. We are not helpless victims, just waiting to be saved by science. We heal ourselves continually. Science is in its infancy when it comes to fully understanding how our brains and bodies work. It is not easy to change our thinking or behavior in our current food environment, flawed common wisdom, and conflicted health advice. Real food is how we directly affect our bodies and our cell metabolism and DNA expression. Healthy food makes healthier cells, and ultimately healthy people.

There is no single supplement or medication that will give us health. It is the cumulative effect of the quality of our food, how much we move, what toxins we have been exposed to, quality of our thoughts, our passions, and our compassion in life. We are all blessed with a unique, special mind and body. We can choose to take simple steps each day to optimize our health.

Notes

1. American Heart Association (2022) "How Much Sugar is Too Much?" https://www.heart.org/en/healthy-living/healthy-eating/eat-smart/sugar/how-much-sugar-is-too-much.

2. USDA "Dietary guidelines for Americans, 2020-2025 Executive Summary", https://www.dietaryguidelines.gov/sites/default/files/2020-12/DGA_2020-2025_ExecutiveSummary_English.pdf.

3. Harvard Health Publishing. (2022). "The Sweet Danger of Sugar" https://www.health.harvard.edu/heart-health/the-sweet-danger-of-sugar

4. Davis, W. (2017). Undoctored, New York, NY: Rondale (Pages 278-287)

5. Heid, M. (2022, August), "The Truth About Fasting and Type 2 Diabetes", https://time.com/6188405/type-2-diabetes-intermittent-fasting/

6. CDC (2020) "Leading causes of death," https://www.cdc.gov/nchs/fastats/leading-causes-of-death.htm.

7. CDC (2022) "What are the risk factors for heart disease?" https://www.cdc.gov/heartdisease/about.htm.

8. Abramson, J. (2022 April 28). "Big Pharma Is Hijacking the Information Doctors Need Most". https://time.com/6171999/big-pharma-clinical-data-doctors/

9. Mercola, J. (2015). Effortless Healing, New York, New York: Harmony Books. (P.10)

References

Bredesen, D. (2017). The End of Alzheimer's Program. New York, New York: Penguin Publishing Group.

Brogan, K. (2016). A Mind of Your Own. New York, NY: Harper Collins Publisher.

Davis, W. (2017). Undoctored. New York, NY: Rondale Inc.

Davis, W. (2012). Wheat Belly. Toronto, Canada: Harper Collins Publishers Ltd.

DiNicolanonio, J. (2017). The Salt Fix. New York, New York: Potter/Ten Speed/Harmony/Rodale.

DiNicolanonio, J. and Fung, J. (2019) The Longevity Solution. Las Vegas: Victory Belt Publishing.

Fung, J and Moore, J. (2016). The Complete Guide to Fasting. Las Vegas, NV: Victory Belt Publishing.

Fung, J (2018). The Diabetes Code. Vancouver/Berkley: Greystone Books Ltd.

Gioffre, D. (2021). Get Off Your Sugar. New York, New York: Hachette Go.

Hyman, M. (2022). Food Fix. New York New York: Little Brown Spark.

Lustig R. (2013). Fat Chance. New York, New York: Penguin Publishing Group.

Lustig R. (2021). Metabolical. New York, New York: Harper Collins Publisher Ltd.

Lustig R. and Yudkin, J. (2017) Pure, White, and Deadly: Penguin UK.

Mercola, J. (2015). Effortless Healing. New York, New York: Harmony Books.

O'Connell, J. (2010). Sugar Nation. New York, New York: Hyperion.

Perlmutter, D. (2015). Brain Maker. MA, Boston: Little Brown & Company.

Perlmutter, D. (2020). Brain Wash. MA, Boston: Little Brown & Company.

Perlmutter, D. (2022). Drop Acid. MA, Boston: Little Brown & Company.

Perlmutter, D. (2018). Grain Brain. MA, Boston: Little Brown & Company.

Taubes, G. (2016). The Case Against Sugar. London, UK: Portobello Books.

Taubes, G. (2008). Good Calories Bad Calories. New York, New York: Anchor Books.

Teicholz, N. (2015). The Big Fat Surprise. New York, N Y: Simon & Schuster.

About the Author

S. T. Gardner received a Bachelor of Science degree, in electrical engineering from the University of Illinois in Chicago, and an Associate's degree in interior design from The Art Institute of Ft. Lauderdale.

Her curiosity led her to investigate human health. In addition to her research, she has taken courses in nutrition science, cognitive health, and neuroscience. She is fascinated by the delicate communication and signaling process between brain cells and how this amazing, intricate and redundant system can optimize our survival and quality of life.

By writing *Our Choices Matter*, she wants to share the good news about our ability to control our own health destiny and be a part of the positive changes needed in the understanding of how our bodies, food choices, and lifestyle are fundamentally connected.